With love

MW00978978

HEALTH 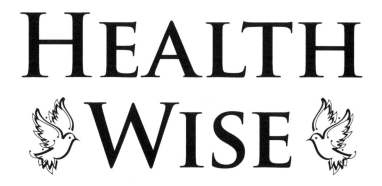 WISE

True Health and Happiness for the Empowered Woman

SUE VAN RAES

BALBOA.
PRESS
A DIVISION OF HAY HOUSE

ISBN: 978-1-4525-5526-3 (sc)
ISBN: 978-1-4525-5525-6 (e)
ISBN: 978-1-4525-5527-0 (hc)

Library of Congress Control Number: 2012912704

Balboa Press books may be ordered through booksellers or by contacting:

Balboa Press
A Division of Hay House
1663 Liberty Drive
Bloomington, IN 47403
www.balboapress.com
1-(877) 407-4847

Printed in the United States of America

Balboa Press rev. date: 08/27/12

Let the wind carry your wise ways
Your forgotten rituals
They are in the dust
Buried with the countless civilizations
They are in the oceans, the salt that licks our wounds
They are in the fire that warms us through and through
They are in the caves that hold our ancestors bones

It is on the wind
Can you not hear her whisper sweetly to you?
It is the last truth of all women
It is the lost truth of all men
It comes from within and without it
It says and replays again and again
This message of welcoming
This message of truth
This message of love
Goddess, sing me home

—unknown

It takes a tribe

Health Wise *is **dedicated***

To my beloved children, Elijah and Ariel, who continually inspire me to live and serve at my highest potential. May your paths continue to be filled with joy, wonder, and beauty.

Thank you

To my parents, who have always been a consistent support in my life, believing in me, and teaching me to open my heart wide and trust.

Thank you.

To my love, Federico, for your limitless devotion, ever- present kindness, and inspirational wisdom. You are what made Health Wise *possible for me. For believing in me even more than I believe in myself.*

Thank you.

To all of my amazing sisters, for always being there for me, through it all, as we venture along all of life's wild ups and downs together.

Thank you.

And of course, to all of the women who have come before me, paved the way for me, shared their stories with me, and opened their hearts in the name of the divine feminine.

Thank you.

And finally, to the divine feminine present in each of us, who wrote this book through me.

Thank you.

CONTENTS

*COVER PHOTO BY D'ANTONIO PHOTOGRAPHY
AND COVER DESIGN BY SOLUA DESIGNS*

FOREWORD

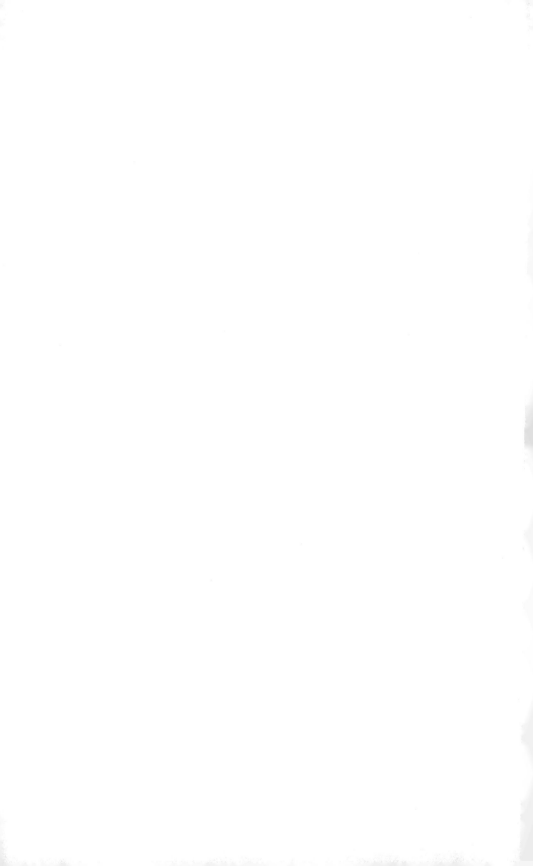

Nine years ago, I made a big decision. I was nearing the end of my graduate work in Chinese Medicine. I had already spent one full year as a clinic intern doing rounds treating an enormous variety of symptoms and conditions. I had treated everything from the common cold to cancer, and I had experienced without a doubt something I had only intuited up to that point: that recovery is indeed possible without the need for surgery or pharmaceuticals. I had also gained lots of respect for the innovations within Western medicine, specifically in the areas of diagnostics and emergency medicine. Yet, despite all of my years of study and clinical experience, something was still missing from the picture.

Medicine, at least the type we are exposed to—whether Western or Eastern—is inherently patriarchal. While I was in school, not only were there no courses or clinics dedicated to women's health, there were also no textbooks, no teachers, and ultimately no focus on women. Interestingly, women make up the majority of the patient demographic in integrative medicine. So why did women get the smallest amount of both academic and practical attention? This mystery plagued me for years, and clarity came only once I took the leap and made my big decision.

My decision was to dedicate my life, my resources, and my free time to the discovery, understanding, and healing of women. It was the decision itself—and the energy that such acts of truth bring with them—that began to unravel for me the mystery behind the lack of information on women's health—one day at a time, one patient at a time. I opened my practice and dedicated every open slot to the treatment of girls and women alone. Nearly every patient walked in with what I like to call a "cover symptom"—and ended up dealing with something else entirely. Usually what we uncovered were deep roots for habits and patterns that were laid down years and years prior by a trauma, a relative's unknowing criticisms, or a belief system she unwittingly inherited at an early age. These old roots had grown branches, and the branches were no longer serving her.

Fast-forward nine years. What do I have to say for my "big decision?" The fact that women's studies and women's health have yet to be given their proper place in the budgets of research and academic institutions is only a mystery for one reason. It is because *we* are a mystery. Women are complex. Our finances are tied to our physical health, our physical health is tied to our emotional fitness, our emotional fitness is tied to our hormonal fluctuations, our hormonal fluctuations are tied to our diets, our diets are tied to our communities, our communities are tied to our relationships, and our relationships are only as strong as we are honest—honest with ourselves and honest with each other. So "fixing" us when something seems off balance isn't as easy as following the formulas that the men of medicine have devised. But the more we understand ourselves, the more we will be understood by others; our doctors, our neighbors, our partners, our parents, and most importantly our children. I have always stood by the philosophy that the biggest gift we can offer our children is knowing and understanding ourselves physically, emotionally, and spiritually so that they need not carry all of the baggage we didn't take care of in our own lives.

I was both honored and thrilled when Sue Van Raes asked me to write the foreword to this book. I've known Sue for seven years now and I have always been in awe of the way she is able to balance self-care, care for her children, and care for her career—all the while overcoming life's obstacles with grace. Sue has a lifetime of experience and wisdom to share. She's been sharing it individually, in group settings, and on exclusive retreats, and now the time has come for her to share her wisdom with all of you.

In this book, Sue has laid out a clear map of all the areas that make up a woman's being. She includes ways to wake up those areas we have neglected, ways to celebrate those areas we are proud of, and ways to practice going deeper and deeper into those areas we are afraid of. From our eating habits to our sexual drives, she leaves no stone unturned because, ultimately, each of these stones need turning. Together they redefine what optimal health really looks like for the empowered woman of the 21st century.

Take the time to read and re-read each chapter. Read especially slowly when you come upon the personal stories Sue has selected to help us really understand how best to access our inner wisdom. Practice what she preaches so that you can break the lineage of old and outdated habits that were handed down to you before you pass them down to your children. Study all the methods she offers to increase your intuition so that you can wake up and stay awake for this beautiful journey called life. Feel the presence of all the women who are on this journey with you, and know that you are supported, understood, and witnessed. More than anything, enjoy. Enjoy these words that will ring so true to your spirit.

Reading this book with an open heart, with a beginner's mind, and with a yearning to learn will allow you to make the absolute most of this life you've been given—and will, in turn, help keep your community of women as healthy as can be. There is no more important work on this planet. May the words in this book reflect the empowered woman you already are and help you model that strength for generations to come.

Liza Pascal, L.Ac.
Coach, The Clarity & Strategy Sessions

INTRODUCTION

Mount the stallion of love and do not fear the path, love's stallion knows the way exactly. With one leap, love's horse will carry you home.

- Rumi

This work has been evolving inside of me for my entire womanhood—it still is, and I believe it forever will be. For a long time, I thought writing and sharing this information with others must mean mastering all of these areas within me personally. Truthfully, that is what I strive for—it is why I get up every morning, and it's what gives me the fire and passion for my life. But I must accept in myself that an exploration such as writing this book truly teaches me and helps me evolve as it penetrates so many layers of my being. I may never feel like a master of this mysterious voyage called womanhood, but this pilgrimage into writing about women, health, and our diverse connections to spirit, love, and higher consciousness fills me. So it may be that this process of writing and exploring is one of my biggest life teachers.

Some would say I wear my heart on my sleeve, some would say I am "sensitive," some would say emotional, spiritual, intense, but truth be known I am simply just me, just as you are you. My life is about working with what I have, making the most of the moment, loving deeply, learning the life lessons that come to me, and sharing more pleasure and joy with more folks than I can even begin to imagine. I have learned that this life is about allowing my own fullest expression, and with each chapter of this book I have undertaken deep, deep inquiry into myself, as well as into womanhood as a whole. I strive to help bring forth a collective energy in which we can all flourish together. I continue to do this work in the name of womanhood, health, and inspiring a path of bliss and empowerment that is sustainable, both for myself and for all of you.

My life has taken many unexpected twists and turns, to which I'm sure many of you can relate. I have learned lessons that I never would have chosen for myself, experienced things I never wanted to experience. I have been pushed to my edge of my suffering, fear and anxiety, as well as to my edge of love and bliss, just as most of us have. I have felt beautiful and radiant like the empress who embodies femininity, unconditional love, and nurturing. I have also endured feelings of inadequacy, unattractiveness, and hopelessness with myself and with the way life felt wrong, backwards, and even downright accidental at times. Life has been, thus far, a rainbow of emotions, but there has always been a light, a fire, a connection to spirit, other women, and especially to the circle of sisters who always pull through for me, supporting, loving, and allowing the space for it all to work its way through to connection with my source, with meaning, and ultimately, to an experience of fulfillment. I will now take the opportunity to thank all of you who have been my sisters—you know who you are. I could never have gotten here alone. You all are my life vest, always keeping me afloat. The hard moments in my life would have felt so much lonelier and more desolate without you. I also want to take this time to acknowledge all of the men in my life, including my two incredible sons, Elijah and Ariel, who have been an amazing reflection for me, always teaching me more about myself. I feel so blessed to be surrounded by good men in my community—men who do their work, walk their talk, and support me in so many ways. I believe men can hold sacred space for women to dance in freedom, sensuality, and our authentic femininity.

I feel lucky to have been touched by so many amazing people. After a traditional family upbringing, hard-core competitive sports, many adventurous travels, marriage, pregnancy, home birth, motherhood, divorce, deep community connection, lots and lots of school, founding my own business, writing, making love, dancing, practicing deep spirituality and ritual, overwhelming financial stress, retreating, living simply and close to the earth, cooking, coaching, therapy, bodywork, depression, moments of total bliss and joy, much deep gratitude, teenagers (they travel in packs and eat a lot), meditation, supportive sisterhood, a lot of yoga, and endless amounts of pleasure, I feel it is finally time to share with others the culmination of my life experience up to this point. At times, it feels like I have done so much personal work that I should have stretch marks, but I am continually fed by my process of looking and listening inward. This work is what inspires me in life.

This book is not really about me, but rather it is about the larger experience of being a woman—a woman with passion. Imagine thriving in every area of your life, and finding a path filled with all that we women generally want in our lives: balance, purpose, inspiration, creativity, love, the list goes on. When we begin to thrive, we begin to feel great about ourselves, and it shows. Imagine if your life felt like it was totally in alignment, from the inside to the outside. WOW!

Here we are entering into this experience together. *Health Wise* is a wanderlust, a personal quest, and an opportunity to invoke your true inner connection and spirit. This quest, a microcosm for every aspect of life, is one that is based on finding pleasure, joy, grace, and inner peace, while breaking free, into our most authentic selves. It is about lifting the masks, so to speak—the masks we wear as we embrace the world, but also the masks we live behind, hiding even from ourselves. *Health Wise* offers empowering work and inspiration that will guide you further down the road to contentment and self-awareness. *Health Wise* unveils the truth of our hearts. Mastering ourselves is a process that can take a lifetime, but somewhere in the midst of all of this growth and wisdom, we start to feel the progress. The reflection we are so used to seeing of ourselves begins to really shift. Our relationships improve, our thoughts improve, our overall happiness and joy increases. We communicate well, we feel and celebrate our successes, our bodies are healthy, vibrant, and resilient, even amidst health challenges, and this personal revolution we have been truly striving for is now taste-able. This is THRIVING.

Each of these chapters will take us on a personal expedition, diving deeper and deeper into ourselves. We will study, understand, reveal, and remember some of the most intimate parts of who we are and what we are here to do on our own personal quests for health and happiness. This journey together is about removing our blocks so our spirit is free to flow through us. *Health Wise* offers practical tools and exercises that can help you see ways to move through life with ease and grace. You will also investigate internal experiences that will rock your world. You will have many breakthroughs, I guarantee. Be prepared to have one of the most amazing experiences of your life. Intend to create a space in which you will stretch out into your full potential of joy and radiance.

One of my passions is to be surrounded by groups of women gathering together in a common vision. I have often participated in and facilitated these kinds of gatherings and groups. I love to guide women on their journeys, leading groups and creating the space for us to come together. The groups I lead have proven to be dynamic and rich and have taught me so much about myself: my edge, my confidence, and my sense of trust in the higher forces that guide us into deeper transformation. The power that women can create when we gather as we tend to each other, as we allow each other to unfold, is a power that is rare in this universe.

As you read through the following pages, you will find many stories, examples, and testimonials that come from real-life experiences that have occurred during, or have been shared at, my workshops and events, as well as in my private practice, in which I work with women as both a nutritionist and a coach.

As my process unfolds, I am blessed to witness more opening and vulnerability, both in myself and in others, as we join together on our path to blissful living. I see magic happening, I see intuition speaking more and more loudly, I see us caring for and nurturing each other in perfect and divine ways. I feel the collective energies profoundly revealing space for true and deep healing to occur.

I feel as we women find our way back home to each other—to the divine feminine, and to our sisters—things begin to align all around us. Energy shifts in large waves, and then we find ourselves with more courage, more trust, and more support to do what it is we are truly called to do here on the planet. To be fully in service to life itself is the truest mission for me, and I hope that, as you read and write and witness yourself through the following pages, you will be inspired, as well. You are invited to find your true calling, and trust yourself enough to move forward. Connect inward with your inherent voice of truth, and then together, let's take the leap!

TRUE HEALTH

Being happy doesn't mean that everything is perfect. It means that you've decided to look beyond the imperfections.

–Marianne Williamson

I t has become so common to hear people talking about health, especially with the booming health trend, and the rise of healthy foods and health-related products that are taking over the consumer marketplace. This seems to be a catchy word making a mark in our society, and yet there is still confusion about what the word *health* actually means, the definition has been expanding, so the word encompasses a great deal more now than it used to. Much of my work has been related to re-creating a strong and pure definition of the word *health* and finally, with the inspiration of many teachers, clients, and friends, I feel as though I have come to clarity in this regard.

During my classes and women's groups, this is one of the primary discussions that we have as we begin our work together. This conversation sets the stage for how we move forward. It is always interesting to go around the room and hear what people have to say. Some are very focused on the physical symptoms, while some are much more focused on the process, the lessons, and the life challenges that have been their biggest teachers.

Some of the most standard definitions of *health* essentially boil down to "the overall condition of the individual." *Health* has been defined as being "a state of complete physical, mental, and social well-being and not merely the absence of disease or infirmity." *Health* is "a resource for everyday life, not the objective of living." *Health* is a positive concept emphasizing both social and personal resources, as well as physical capacities. In many Western medical interpretations, *health* is thought of as simply "the absence of disease."

There are so many ways to define and relate to one's own health. But I pose this question to you: What does *true health* mean to you? What do you want your health to look like, and feel like, and how do you intend to reach those personal health goals? Where have you been in your relationship with your health, and where are you going? These are all questions we will dive into in the following chapters. Here we are just planting the seeds, and beginning to look inward to find all the inspiration we need to begin a meaningful path together.

HYGEIA

Hygeia is the Greek goddess who was said to watch over the health of the people of ancient Athens. Her healing power lay not with surgery and medication, but with education and healthy living. She taught that healing is both a personal choice and a personal commitment. Being empowered meant tuning into one's own body, learning what works, what aggravates symptoms, and what nourishes one's own body, mind, and spirit. That is where true healing was believed to be possible.

Health Wise takes this approach and begins to return health to its rightful place: the hands of individuals, empowering each of us to listen, to pay attention, and to use our intuition and wisdom, and to guide us down a road to greater health and freedom. As we refine our relationships with ourselves, we are closer to listening and knowing how to maintain this inner and outer balance that keeps us aligned with health and our own healing potential, leaving us feeling more empowered than ever.

IN SICKNESS AND IN HEALTH

One question that I often ponder is: Can you be healthy if you are sick? As we know there are always ailments, health challenges, and stress challenges in our individual experiences, along with the collective state of health in our society. Our bodies constantly express different emotions and experiences in the physical form as an expression of our state of inner health and the connection between our minds and bodies. Our health is not a constant, but rather, a wave of reflection of our inner truth that is always unfolding before us.

I believe that health is not limited to our physical symptoms, but is also about how we relate to our symptoms. How is your self talk? Are you fear-based? Are you strong and positive? Are you looking at the whole picture, or are you focused on just the physical manifestation? Are you looking at all the different areas in our lives, keeping balance, purpose, inspiration, healthy relationships, managed stress levels, and healthy inner dialogue? This, to me, is a deeper reflection of our complete true health and well-being. The inner listening and outer expression we experience together create a true, moment-to-moment, live expression of our holistic health.

Whenever there is total alignment from the inside out there is no problem, no conflict. Why are we so often lacking this alignment? Normally we want several things at once. We want to be healthy, lose weight, feel vital and alive, sleep well, and look radiant. Of this we are often quite conscious. But somehow our inner strength and will don't fully support our ideal outer manifestation of health. We often know what we need to do or change, yet we get stuck in the process of keeping our commitment to ourselves, and have trouble finding and maintaining self-control and diligence. We give our power away to our weaknesses, addictions, or old patterns, and then often give up altogether. This model of seeking greater health and happiness is outdated, and not very functional. It poses too much conflict between our willpower and our temptations. Caring for our health requires vision, wisdom, and a true knowing of what we really want and need, so that we can begin to fuel our health with a sense of purpose, determination, and diligence, and finally get out of our own way.

DEFINING HEALTH

Before we go any further, it is important to establish our language and definition of terms. As mentioned earlier, our definition of "health" has become so ambiguous that at this point we might as well be shooting in the dark. To unveil what we really want, we need to start with what "health" actually means to each of us! It is important to do this work for yourself, and find your own definition.

To get you started, here are some ways I like to define "health":

- Health is our mind/body experience of being in the world.

- Health is the way we relate to, feel in, think about, and move our bodies.

- Health is the intricate balance of our inner experience and our outer expression.

- Health is the way we relate to our day-to-day challenges, pains, sickness, stress, and joy.

- Health is the way we give and receive love, the way we communicate, our attitudes toward our work in the world, the way we talk to the people who are close to us, and the way we take care of ourselves.

- Health is the quality of our emotional experience on the inside.

It is true that our health does take some inner work and inquisition—in yoga there is a word, *svadhaya*, or self-study, which can mean the practice of learning about the self. As women, all the layers we live through influence each other. This is why our health is not a linear entity, but more or a mysterious unveiling of each of our individual whole selves. I believe that our creation of health begins with the seed of desire to know ourselves deeply. When we unveil our clear vision of what health means to us, and what that looks like specifically, this vision will propel us forward. This is far stronger than willpower, far superior to an outdated paradigm that dis-empowers our intuition and inner wisdom. Health begins with reflection, understanding, and the creation of what it is that we want for ourselves. This is the commitment, but an easier one to stick with because it is one that speaks the truth of our heart.

As we move into the following chapters, remember, this is an in-depth inquiry into our whole life experience. It's a chance to find out more about the sense of health we feel and know (or *don't* feel and know) in every area of our lives. This is a chance for you to see where you "have it down" and also to uncover the shadows, or the places that do not align with your highest self and your greatest health potential. Once we uncover these more challenging areas, you will see that sometimes just by shining the light of awareness on them, change can and will begin to happen. Simply by shifting our attention and our intention in various ways, we experience transformation.

MEET ANGELA:

Angela is one of my long-time clients. She recently shared with me that nowadays it's easy for her to prioritize and maintain vibrant health. But it hasn't always been this way...

Angela lives in Denver, Colorado, and works as an engineer, a yoga instructor, and now a facilitator of cleanse programs for yoga studios across the country. When she was only 21, she was diagnosed with an "incurable" autoimmune disease called interstitial cystitis, which left her feeling helpless, confused, and experiencing severe pain and terribly low energy. But somewhere deep inside she knew that the diagnosis of her illness as "incurable" did not have to be true for her. She sought out many alternative healers and wise teachers, such as acupuncturists, nutritionists, yoga teachers, psychics, and reiki healers. With a deep sense of trust in her inner guidance, Angela did a lot of work around how to find balance in her life and create habits of clean living. As she dove deeper into purification, whole foods, and the mind-body approach to healing and cleansing, she found that her symptoms were diminishing.

After a few years of steadily growing in strength, and caring for her health intuitively, she was able to minimize her symptoms until they were virtually non-existent. Angela has been symptom-free for almost 10 years now, and is an inspiration to others, sharing the message that your health is up to you, and coaching and guiding others on their healing journeys. During one of the meetings of our recent year-long women's health group in which she participated she said, "If you listen and follow what your higher self guides you to, keeping all the little pieces in balance, you can find a peaceful health experience, even in the face of supposedly incurable illness."

Nurturing her health now feels easy to Angela because of the cumulative effects of her commitment to heal, and her ability to follow her own intuition in doing so. Her mantra throughout all the years was: "I will get better, I will do whatever it takes." She believes this commitment also helped her attract the healers and teachers that she needed.

Angela participated in my year-long women's group to help her continue to connect with community, heal some of the wounds from her experience of her autoimmune disease, and dig deeper into the underlying thoughts and beliefs that lay underneath the health struggles she had faced.

In her work as a health coach and yoga instructor, Angela listens for commitment in others as a powerful tool to support their healing. She also emphasizes the importance of practice, persistence, and patience—celebrating the small successes, and working to stay on track.

Here are some of the practices that were part of Angela's healing process, many of which she still uses regularly to help her stay on track:

- *Cleansing*
- *Yoga*
- *Nutritional education*
- *Acupuncture*
- *Chiropractic*
- *Energy healing (Barbara Brennan style)*
- *Massage*
- *Craniosacral therapy*

DAILY REGIMEN

- *Daily meditation practice*
- *Eating well*
- *Pharmaceutical grade supplementation*
- *Regular upkeep with healer (once or twice per month)*

Angela says: "Life is cyclical, and with either traumatic injury or chronic illness, you could be struggling in one way but the rest of you is feeling great. Your emotions could be weighing you down but you could be empowered by how your healing is progressing and feeling strong in the face of whatever comes your way. You have to focus on the positive."

MEET DONNA:

Donna is a dancer, lover of intellectual activities, and psychology graduate. She was diagnosed with MS 18 years ago, and she spends her days mothering her daughter, Maya, and working from home, where she is able to pace herself.

Donna is now 46 years old and says she is feeling healthier and more vibrant than she has in years

Donna shared with me that, when working outside the home, she was dependent on others' schedules and rhythms, which didn't always work for her.

She has learned that lowering her standards in terms of the amount she can do physically, listening to what she actually can do and being okay with that—not being extreme—is a path to true health.

Donna is inspired by both pleasure and function. "Enjoying the things that my body can do, and using my body to do what it can do in the world—I have learned not to take it for granted!" She has lost and regained function so many times that she has had to learn to appreciate the capabilities of her body.

"My body is always changing. I had related to myself as a thin, strong dancer, and then became someone who felt fat and out of shape, then eating disorders, being ill, being injured. At 46, I am feeling better about my body than I ever have before.

Working with Sue's women's group gave me an amazing support system. This is not a job I want to do alone.

The group is an important and valuable circle of people who became 'our women,' where we could touch in and go deeper, and had permission to be real. This became my place to be radically honest and to not have to be 'fine' all the time. What an important reflection of being healthy: authenticity."

Donna says that creating a really nice environment that she loves to spend time in, resting and being healthy, is also very important to her. She created sacred space around and inside her house and gardens. Particularly because she was bedridden in her home two different times, for two years each time, her house became her healing space and it was therefore crucial that that space feel good to her.

"I have learned that being okay being with myself so I can slow down and be present—not run away—helps me. Being overly busy was a running away mechanism. I believe in order to find balance and true health there has to be a level of being okay being settled in body and mind. Health, for me, also includes my relationship to food—eating really well. I love using cooking as a primary creative element, and also a way to connect with family more deeply."

Donna believes you can find health even amidst serious health challenges, and considers herself healthier now than she ever was before her MS diagnosis.

"Being sick profoundly changed my life. I have let go of many things, but also gained so many, leaving me with a healthier balance overall. MS has taught me so much about being healthy."

HOME PRACTICE

Journal Exercise

1.   *Journal Question*

*Sit down in a quiet space and get comfortable. Give yourself a timed 15-minute session of brainstorming to allow your subconscious mind to meet your conscious mind on paper. Write down anything and everything that **"true health"** means to you—no boundaries, no rules, just you and your pen. Be free to express without judgment. This is a chance to let it all out—the good and the bad—and create material to reflect upon, learn about yourself, and clear out the thoughts and beliefs that no longer serve you. This material will guide you to our next exercise.*

Note: Watch for any old belief systems, ideas, emotional blocks, or breakthroughs.

2.   *Creating the Health You Want*

Looking back at the journal exercise, begin to make a list for yourself that reflects what you want for your overall health, your vision of health for yourself. Place this list somewhere where you will read it often, such as your fridge, your nightstand, or a place where you do spiritual practices, such as an altar. Read it daily with intention and vigor.

Suggested Affirmation

"My health belongs to me. I am an advocate for my own health. I am making healthy choices today that will enable me to achieve TRUE HEALTH in a sustainable, positive way."

INTERNAL
AWAKENING

SECRET #1
On-Purpose

I say, follow your bliss and don't be afraid, and doors will open where you didn't know they were going to be.

—Joseph Campbell

Tell your heart that the fear of suffering is worse than the suffering itself. And no heart has ever suffered when it goes in search of its dream.

—Paulo Coelho

The word **purpose** comes from the Latin word meaning *"to put forth."* The literal definition is "action serving to change the state of conditions in a given environment, usually to one with a perceived better set of conditions or parameters from the previous state." Yes, the action and intention to create! Purpose is the action or vision we put forth.

When I think of what I intend to "put forth" into the world, I grapple with the same predicament that many of us face: "How do I put forth my self, my heart, my will in this world, and how do I uncover these qualities in myself? How do I create my path to living on-purpose with clarity, distinction, and assertiveness?

Some common complaints from women are: "I don't know what I want," or "I can't seem to find my passion or purpose," or "I am on the wrong path and I don't know how I got here." I believe that we can so often get caught up in what is going on around us, in our partners' lives, our children's lives, or our mothers' lives, that we put everyone else's well-being ahead of our own, and before we know it we have lost our own sense of self. We can easily give little parts of ourselves away until one day we wake up and we don't recognize who we are anymore. Now I don't want to take away from the fact that women are amazingly nurturing beings in general. We can take care, tend to, and hold the space for other beings to flourish. But what I am talking about is women finding a way to truly live with purpose and intention, and to fulfill the deepest parts of ourselves, which includes having a thriving relationship and healthy family, as well as enjoying our own individual spiritual heart awakening that supports us as we joyfully live all the roles that we play.

Living with purpose feels like freedom from the inside out. Purpose gives us a sense of passion in each day--it wakes us up in the morning excited to get out of bed, ready to be in our lives fully. Living with purpose isn't always an easy undertaking, but it is one that will not only serve us as individuals, but will also serve our families, communities, and colleagues.

You see, when we are "stuck" in our lives, or unsure of how to live on-purpose, we can end up feeling depleted. Our energy is not able to move freely through us, and we feel drained, lethargic, and sluggish about life. Life becomes a big chore that never ends, like an endless to-do list (we all know what that is like!), and we feel like we are swimming upstream. Can you relate?

When we are living a life of purpose, we feel clear, energized, and creative, and we experience a well of energy that enlivens us, creating radiance, vitality, and bliss. Sounds good, right? Where do I sign up?

Well, for some of us our purpose is obvious and clear, and it is accessible. It takes but a moment to define, and we are confident we are on the path. For others, though, it feels like a mountain that we will never be able to climb, or maybe never even find the trail map for! What can we do to learn more about how to uncover this idea, this vision, this well of creativity called purpose that is inherently present in each of us, ready to be unleashed like a wild animal? It is there—yes it is! Somehow, somewhere along the way, we just lose it for a while sometimes. Now it is time to remember.

The reason we all crave living a life with vision and purpose is because when we are living this way, a true expression of ourselves is being born. We are living the fullest expression of ourselves. Have you ever met someone who inspires you, who you look up to? What is it about this person that pulls you in? You see, it is our sacred commitment to ourselves to figure out our purpose out in this life. It is our deepest yearning and deepest longing to feel the inner freedom that living with purpose and vision bring us. We just have to commit to spending the time and energy to remember sooner rather than later. We spend so much time in this Western culture waiting for the external situation to line up just right, for it to be the right time—waiting, waiting, and more waiting. What are we waiting for again?

Waiting for a train to go,
or a bus to come, or a plane to go
or the mail to come, or the rain to go
or the phone to ring, or the snow to snow
or waiting around for a Yes or a No
or waiting for their hair to grow.
Everyone is just waiting.
Waiting for the fish to bite
or waiting for wind to fly a kite
or waiting around for Friday night
or waiting, perhaps, for their Uncle Jake
or a pot to boil, or a Better Break
or a string of pearls, or a pair of pants
or a wig with curls, or Another Chance.
Everyone is just waiting.
NO!
That's not for you!
Somehow you'll escape
all that waiting and staying.
You'll find the bright places
where Boom Bands are playing.

—Dr. Seuss

One of my teachers has a saying that often reminds me to get my butt in gear, so to speak:

"This is not a dress rehearsal."

This really says it all to me. When I hear this quote, which now lives in my own head, I tend to get moving, find my action-oriented goals and intentions, open to all that I can create, find my fearlessness, and take the leap.

You see, we are creatures of habit. We humans love to make excuses, avoid parts of ourselves, and even turn the face of denial towards whatever reality is confronting us. We can easily spend years making excuses about why not to put ourselves, and our vision and purpose first. In my women's groups, this is always the most prevalent limiting factor. Just getting those women through the door, taking the time to commit to their process and showing up at group for themselves, is easier said than done. I so often hear about the kids, about the guilt they feel doing something just for themselves, spending money on themselves, or having to have Dad babysit. As women, living our purpose can fall so far down the list of priorities that we often can't even find it at the end of the day. We get buried in the other parts of life that are important. But if we are living with a strong vision and purpose, the amount we can get done in a day and the amount of energy we have left for all of our other roles is remarkably higher.

YOUR SACRED RIGHT

How would it feel if you were told that it is your sacred right as a human being to not only discover your purpose, but to actually live with purpose every day of your life? If you were to clear away all the other worries, blocks, and obligations and simply believe that your purpose is your divinity, and that it can and will permeate every role, and every part of your day-to-day. To me this idea feels like a great big exhale. Phew.

In our Western culture we are so often taught that living from our purpose is almost selfish or impractical, as if we should decide to move forward with decisions that make the most "sense," practically speaking, and ignore what is truly wanting to emerge. I was recently reading some teachings from Deepak Chopra in which he tells a story about his children and how he raised them to always honor their individual gifts in the world. He taught them not to worry about grades, money, or success, but only to focus on what it is they have to offer the world within their purpose and service. He said he would always take care of them, and they could fully live out their purpose without all the added financial pressures most of us feel. As it turned out, his children always got excellent grades and grew up into very successful adults who did not need to be supported by him. He gave them permission to live with purpose, and everything else aligned for them from there.

With the recent turn in the economy, I was challenged financially for a few months. I was questioning my job, my career, and whether or not I would "make it," so to speak. At one point I had a realization that I needed to connect with my purpose, and remembered that if I lived from there it would all work out, as the universe promises to always work that way. I would often wake up in the middle of the night and begin to panic, but I would catch myself and remember: "purpose, purpose, purpose . . . , " and things would gradually subside into a feeling of trust and faith. What a relief!

This work has changed my life forever, and I will continue to share it with others on my journey, as we all need a chance to rediscover the importance of living this way. Living with purpose impacts our health, our parenting, our relationships, and our overall experience of joy each and every day.

HOW DO I FIND MY PURPOSE?

Uncovering who you truly are can sometimes feel like finding a needle in a haystack. With all of our paradigms and beliefs working and weaving together (which we will talk about later at much greater length in Secret #3) sometimes we are totally blocked, stuck, or depressed. I had a client in one of my groups who said many times, "I have realized that I am on the wrong f$*@ing path!" For the purposes of our discussion here, we'll call her Helen. Her life was not working, her relationship was falling apart, and she felt paralyzed by fear, financial stress, and the thought of being alone. Each time we would gather, this would be her update. No movement, just her soul shriveling up. She is not alone. Many women feel stuck, not only internally/emotionally, but also externally in the situations in which they find themselves, and without the confidence of purpose, it is hard to move forward. After a lot of intention work, a lot of support, and room to go through all the lessons associated with her challenges, Helen did come out on the other side. It took a while--a couple of years in fact--but life supported her, and she shifted into a really powerful place. She is now doing better than ever!

PERSONAL MOTIVATION

I do believe that we all have specific gifts and talents, and are wired for life in individual ways. We can just lose sight of the truth of ourselves. If you think back to yourself as a child, who were you? What were you known for; what did you hear your parents, friends, and teachers saying about you? What did you want to be; who did you want to be? The reason I ask is because our essence moves through many stages as we age, but it doesn't actually change much overall. The way we were as a child, the way we moved through life back then may have been young, but it was also most often not as clouded by negative beliefs. Maybe we loved animals, babies, dancing, or art. Maybe we were known to be really funny, dedicated and determined, or maybe quiet and introspective. I remember my family always talking about my focus as a gymnast, and my love for food and cooking. So it's interesting that I became a nutritionist, yogini, and life coach. My family, of course, was not surprised. What was **your** very favorite thing to do as a young person?

My son's class did a unit on heroes last year. They all had to pick a hero, study why this person was heroic, and break down the work this hero did into qualities or a purpose that the hero embodied. All the parents got to join together to witness our children dress up like their heroes and act out a short interview; then we all shared about our own personal heroes who speak to our hearts, and why. I thought it was a great exercise in looking deeply at the qualities that heroes embody and that inspire us—qualities like strength, determination, positive thinking, and being of service to those in need, or inspiring large groups of people. If you were to name your own hero, who would it be, and why? Or if you already have a hero, who is it, and what makes him or her your hero? What part of you can you nurture to grow those same heroic seeds in yourself? There is a great worksheet for this on the Health Wise website for you to work with. www.HealthWise-Woman.com/purpose ♀

PERSONAL OBSTACLES TO ACKNOWLEDGE

Reconnecting with your purpose as an adult is truly possible, but often can come with many obstacles, including old, ineffective thought patterns and beliefs. The very things that have blocked you up to this point will likely stand out loud and clear as you start to befriend your purpose. Stay strong, be the witness, and move forward with awareness when fears come up, when negative beliefs tell you that you can't, and when you watch yourself make excuses in your life.

FEAR OF FAILURE

The fear of failure or inadequacy can often turn us away from moving into purposeful living. It can feel like the challenge is too much. But once we uncover our purpose, we have a sacred contract with ourselves to **fulfill** it. Wow, that's a big commitment. Maybe it is "safer" to stay in the dark? If we have chosen to stay in the dark so far, it's like a 180-degree flip to live from purpose. I mean, what would happen if, after all of the work you went through finding your purpose, you then witnessed your life falling apart? Finally identifying our purpose, but then not feeling able to create a life infused with it, can be heartbreaking. All of these fears are totally real. The good news is: I believe that as we identify our fears, they become more and more powerless. If fear is just energy, then it may be that all we need to do is face our fears, look them straight in the eye, and begin to use the strength of our inner purpose to move forward.

ADDICTION TO OUR OWN SUFFERING

One common way we block ourselves from our inherent bliss, purpose, and fulfillment is related to the addictions most of us have to negative thoughts and beliefs, and to our own suffering. For many of us, sitting in our own suffering (large or small) is a pattern that has formed and become a habitual way we move through life! It is crazy how our minds work. Where do you embellish your own suffering? What do you get from it? In some twisted way we all "get something" out of complaining, being depressed, or playing the victim. Maybe we get more attention, maybe we get to be "lazy," or maybe we are simply used to feeling this way, so this state has become the place where we feel most comfortable. What do you get out of it? Inquire into your own patterns with suffering, and take a closer look. Things may not change right away, but at least you will be more aware of your patterns, and be able to witness them more objectively. Eventually it can become almost comical to see these patterns and learn where you give into them. They may have started in your childhood, in a relationship, or even in a hard phase of your life. There are many opportunities for these patterns to become a habit, but just as many opportunities to change them with love and awareness.

CHECK IN OR CHECK OUT

Self-soothing is a high priority in our self-care, but "checking out" is a different thing, and it means shutting down, turning a blind eye, or avoiding feeling or experiencing the strong emotions that we may be afraid of (including bliss, for some). If the pattern of "checking out" is a big one for you, manifesting in addiction, denial, or dissociation, taking gradual steps toward healing is important. You may consider appropriate therapies to find the best plan to change the behavior to something that does serve you. It is challenging to live with purpose when you have addictive patterns blocking your progress. Now don't get me wrong, we all have these patterns, it just depends on where yours fall on the spectrum of self-destruction. Alcoholism, drug addiction, or any behavior that endangers your physical or emotional safety should be addressed with a lot of care and even, in many cases, professional help. I find having a friend or support of some kind that is in place to call when strong feelings arise to help remind you about your higher purpose and what you really want for yourself is critical and very effective. Having accountability in place makes all the difference. This is why AA and similar groups are so effective for so many people. Learning how to give strong emotions the space to move through you, and the voice they need to speak their message to you, is going to help your process of self-discovery progress more quickly.

THE POWER OF INTENTION

One of the first steps toward living a life infused with purpose is to take the essence of all the other practices covered in this book, and begin to weave these ideas into our lives through vision and intention. The question is, how connected are you to your own inner voice or source energy, and how often can you remember to reconnect, remaining clear, open, and energetic? As you practice keeping this connection, your purpose and vision will flow through you more easily, more abundantly, and more freely.

Returning to yourself, and allowing you and the truth of you to emerge, is the way to let your purpose come through. You can simply **intend** to live with purpose, and this in itself carries a lot of potential energy along with it.

Sometimes, it is helpful to do some journaling using a leading sentence format such as

"Life inspires me when I am

_____."

Trusting that we are in the right place at the right time and that there are no mistakes, or wrong decisions, helps us along. Remembering our essence along the path to purpose and passionate living is the foundation of this work.

VISIONING

I like to think of visioning as a chance to make a "conscious plan" that we can then carry out in every area of life. You know that life is going to continue happening whether you are conscious or unconscious, so why not have a plan that suits you? Why not make the choices, look at where you need to grow and thrive, and set up the structures that will support you on your path to more blissful living? It is a question of being in the driver's seat of your own life versus just seeing where you end up if you let someone else drive the car without asking where it's headed.

Once you have the essence of your purpose moving, and your vision is pouring out of you, notice the ways in which you are beginning to create the life you want. Notice the ways in which you are aligned and in gratitude for the gifts, whether they are always the way you expect and desire, or not. Soon, you will begin to see the divine process of living with intention, as the little shifts you make become obvious, as the right opportunities present themselves, and you find yourself living in deeper alignment with your authentic truth. The organic process by which opportunities appear can barely be grasped by the human mind. The vision is the part we can control, create, and be inspired about!

REFINING YOUR SKILLS

For example, if you see yourself giving back to the environment and teaching others eco-conscious living, you may need to hone your public speaking or grant-writing skills. You may want to learn how to use social media and blogging as ways to connect with others and share your valuable information.

You may know people who inspire you in your field, who you would like to have mentor you, and you may notice that you do well learning experientially with the continued support of a role model.

You may notice that you start to shift the messages that you send to your family at home, by restructuring the shopping to a more eco-friendly approach, by adjusting your children's chores to involve more eco-products and more mindfulness for the environment, and by shifting the outings you choose to share with your family to ones that benefit the environment, like biking together to events instead of driving. This alone may reinvigorate your home life, as well as your relationship with your husband or partner.

How does your purpose infuse every area of your life?

Your purpose is deeper than what you do for work, or what roles you play each day, and more about why you want to play those roles, and how they are tailored to, and inspiring for you.

POSITIVE STRUCTURES

Who can support you in this process?

We all have days when we run out of steam, or when our self-doubt kicks in, so be sure that you are set up with the right support systems to help you through these times. I just requested that my financial coach set up a group of entrepreneurial women to support each other in our financial goals. I know I can do it alone, but with the support of this group of like-minded peers, and a leader who is knowledgeable and inspiring, I know that I will truly thrive. Read more about this in Secret #7: Vibrant Health, Vibrant Wealth.

Living with purpose and intention is a path that I believe feels good to all of us. Feeling "integrity" with ourselves, and with our connection to source energy and our heart's truth is what brings us fulfillment in our lives. It is there, available to you, and ready to be freed in you when you decide and open to it and stand centered in your true self around your purpose. There may be obstacles along the way, but remember they are your teachers. They help you to see more clearly, and reflect back to you where you need to unveil more of you.

To me, purpose is our guiding light that helps us trust our path, knowing this is the best way for us—that our journey is moving along and creating perfect harmony and balance for our gifts to emerge and our hearts to be expressed in the world.

"When you dance, your purpose is not to get to a certain place on the floor. It's to enjoy each step along the way."

—Wayne Dyer

HOME PRACTICE

1.   *Life inspires me when I am*

_____ .

Write out this statement 10 times. See what comes.

2.   *Hero study: Who are your heroes, and what heroic qualities do you value in them? How can you infuse your life with more of these qualities? What skills do you need to do so? Visit the Health Wise Website for exciting downloads around the hero study.* www.HealthWise-Woman.com/purpose ♀

3.   *Create Vision Board infused with your purpose* (more on HealthWise-Woman.com/purpose)

MEET PAIGE

Paige is a 23-year-old college student who has been working with me for the past year. Paige loves playing sports, writing poetry, studying chemistry, and participating in community-related activities.

Paige has done something that's quite common among young people living under the pressure of heavy-duty college studies: she has begun to lose herself, forgetting to create time for her passions. She often goes into an "autopilot" mode that feels empty and uninspiring. Working together, Paige and I helped her connect more and more to a sense of purpose in her life so she could feel more connected to herself and her passions as she completed her last year of college.

Paige describes her work around purpose as "creating intention around being aware, and riding out the full course" of any action that she takes. Diving into this purpose inquiry has helped her realize how to engage in what she wants more fully.

Paige shares:

"Sharing my purpose with people is key. Make yourself responsible by bringing it out into the social realm.

I feel internally driven towards a sense of harmony and balance. Whenever I feel that, I feel happy. Infusing my life with purpose makes me the most capable and effective person I could imagine being.

This whole process has been a rediscovery. Purpose is an integral part of my personality. I had lost sight of meaning and had lost my belief that meaning was real, or that I could invest any faith in it at all. I had questions around my identity and where the driving force was for a meaningful life."

Paige believes that putting purpose in a new context comes from an internal well that helps you continue on with the work, rather than from an external source of motivation. She strives to keep harnessing this as she moves forward, and says, "If we base our existence in this purposeful place, and from here we create beauty, as an active pursuit, we can tap inward with more wisdom, more awareness, and the ability to have the faith to discern the difference."

The essential components that fuel Paige:

- *Music/dance*
- *Writing—mostly poetry*
- *Mutual relationships with people*

From Paige: "In the past, my inspiration and connection to purpose has been very momentary, like reading a quotation, or reading someone's inspiring words. Now it has become important for me to keep inspirations broad and remember to create a collaboration of self-expression in my daily life. Taking responsibility for creating and maintaining day-to-day inspiration for myself is the ticket . . ."

SECRET #2

Food and Freedom

We don't want to EAT hot fudge sundaes as much as we want our lives to BE hot fudge sundaes. We want to come home to ourselves.

- Geneen Roth

W hen it comes to how we relate to food, health, and self-nourishment, there are many challenges of living in the Western world where we are faced with an overload of processed food, health-related issues, the rise of degenerative disease, negative media input, and overall disconnection from our intuition. How can we cultivate more self-love, nutritional wisdom, gentleness, and compassion in our relationship with food?

The practice of ahimsa, included as part of the 8 limbs of yoga, meaning compassion towards the self and others, is a practice that I find can speak directly to the cultivation of a healthy path in our personal relationships with food. Though there are as many relationships with food as there are people on the planet, in the Western world it seems as though a select few remain predominant. Intuitive eating and nutritional wisdom, or rather, the lack thereof, are a source of much stress and inner conflict for many women nationwide. Some of us use food as comfort, some as self-punishment, some of us have compulsive eating patterns, and some of us remain totally disconnected from our eating, the sources of our food, and the primary ways in which we nourish ourselves. Many of us struggle with body image issues, weight management, and even eating disorders, all of which leave us feeling a true lack of self-acceptance, self-love, and self-nourishment. These challenges make it almost impossible to feel the freedom, health, and bliss in our day-to-day lives that we all so desire and deserve. We all know how food can be a source of physical and emotional nourishment, but in practice, we also know that our relationships with food (like all relationships!) can be wrought with challenges and struggles.

Our everyday health practices and goals bring us deeper awareness, a stronger sense of ourselves, and more compassion for ourselves and others. Knowing this, how can we apply these principles to our personal relationships with food? We are essentially looking to guide ourselves back home to our own health, intuition, balance, pleasure, and inner freedom through one of our most primary relationships.

As you read through the following six keys to food and freedom, note that you are being given a road map that paves the way for you to find success and health in your day-to-day food choices, and in relation to your personal psychology around food. These six keys work most effectively when followed in sequence, as skipping one could result in the next one not working as well. The goal here is to provide both the information you need to be informed around your choices and the strategies that you'll likely need to help you implement those choices. For many, healing around food is a winding and complex road. You are not alone. There is a lot of support for you in the upcoming pages, and also on the Health Wise website. We need community and collective wisdom to shift a food paradigm that has been a challenge for women for decades. Please use the resources provided, as they have been tested by many, many women, and have proven to be extremely effective over time when applied with patience and persistence. As you begin to refine and redefine your relationship with food and clarify how to best fuel your sacred body, you will find that you can live life more effectively, be in fuller expression of yourself, and walk through your days with more grace and joy, serving your world more effectively. Our personal work with food psychology is a porthole into the way we relate to our bodies, our challenges, and some of our primary relationships. This important mission, to help heal the feminine when it comes to food, body, and soul, is a critical component in the healing of the feminine.

KEY #1: SIMPLIFY - PURIFY

Just as many of our common daily practices, such as the classical yoga *asanas* (postures) or the ancient meditation practices passed down from the time of the Buddha, stem from age-old traditions and ancient teachings that purify the body, mind, and spirit, so, too, do the most powerful principles of eating. Some of the wise, age-old traditions from cultures far and wide have laid a strong foundation that can help us navigate the jungle of choices we encounter in a way that feels clear and empowering. Many traditions root back to local, whole food-based eating aligned with the seasons. Choosing simple, pure, clean, and natural foods are some of the best guidelines to follow.

Simplify your diet

Eating a simple, whole-food diet rich in fresh fruits, vegetables, high-quality lean protein (animal-based or vegetarian), nuts, seeds, and good oils, such as coconut, olive, and flax, is the first key to resetting our systems, and purifying our bodies. Through this process we are able to get our cravings under control, connect with the seasonal approach to eating, and reset our system as a whole. This approach is not about deprivation, but more about inspiration. When we are inspired about the quality of our food, our health, and the experiences we have in our bodies, we are more likely to feel intuitive and at our highest vitality overall. The consciousness that comes with knowing where our food was grown, who grew it, or where it was raised is yet another way to feel healthy and empowered around our food choices.

What is a whole food?

A whole food is one that is found in nature, without an ingredient list, and usually without a package. The more locally and seasonally we can buy our food, the more nutrient dense and the better. Eating whole foods also inevitably promotes compassion toward the world around us. This, our original way of eating as a species, keeps us in tune with nature, the seasons, and our bodies' true needs for nourishment, which are so often unmet in a typical Western diet of fast food, processed food, and food that resembles nothing natural at all.

Eating whole foods will also provide a foundation to keep our diets pure, nutrient dense, and detoxifying. Cravings will diminish, authentic taste experiences will return, and our body's natural senses of satiation will be more easily available and recognizable, the way they were designed to be.

Breaking Down the Food Groups

Lean Proteins

Lean Proteins are a primary foundation for a healthy metabolism, a strong body, and an abundance of lean muscle mass. So many people in modern-day society are stuck on the sugar/carb roller coaster, and are not getting enough lean protein for their metabolic type and body weight. Without enough protein, we are left dipping into our reserves, sapping our adrenal glands, and depleting our systems. Without the proper amount of lean protein, our bodies have a hard time staying in the fat-burning zone, and we often end up tired, low energy, often nutrient-deficient, and even depressed. The amino acids that create many of our feel-good neurotransmitters are found in lean protein, and are then converted by the digestion and the brain to build serotonin, GABA, and dopamine, keeping us balanced, happy, joyful, and calm.

Be sure that you are mindful of the source of your protein. Because of the processing of meats, and the unethical practices that are prevalent in the meat industry as a whole, it is beneficial to get any animal protein in its most natural, and ethically sound state. Grass-fed beef, free-range chicken and eggs, wild fish that is low in PCB's and heavy metals, whey protein that is low-temperature pasteurized and from grass-fed cows, and soy products that are organic, fermented, and non-GMO are some recommendations. Watch for hormones found in mainstream meat products, as they can really affect a female's hormone balance at any age, and especially during puberty and menopause. Nitrates are best avoided, as they are carcinogenic and toxic to the digestion. Stick with natural, whole, lean, organic proteins whenever possible.

You can download an ideal recommended whole-food list on the Health Wise website: www.HealthWise-Woman.com/foodandfreedom ♀

Natural Fats

As times change, so do our theories around fat, fat-free, and low-fat foods. Foods that used to be considered better choices, we are now informed, can actually be dangerous to our health. How are we to know what is what in the world of fats?

The fat-free era captured the interest of many in our Western population. The campaigns designed to trick us into thinking fat made us fat did not seem all that far-fetched. But through reviewing many case studies, and examining the effects of the fat-free diet, it is now clear to the majority of the health-care industry that this type of diet is detrimental to one's health.

Fats are a very important source of energy in our diets. They are building blocks for many of the hormones and hormone-like substances that our bodies need to function. Without fats in our meals, our bodies lack a natural way of slowing down the feeling of hunger, whilst balancing the primary metabolic hormone, insulin. Many of our fat-soluble vitamins, such as vitamins A, D, E, and K, are transported along with these fats. Many dietary fats also play an important role in the absorption of minerals, the enzymatic breakdown of foods, and the feeling of total nourishment and satisfaction after eating.

Deciding which types of fats to include in your diet is an important consideration. We are bombarded by a variety of fats. It takes some nutritional knowledge to know how to balance the different types of fats, and which ones to stay away from.

Let's examine some of the different types of fats and how they each work in the body:

Saturated fats: A fatty acid becomes a saturated fat, when all of its available carbon bonds are occupied by a hydrogen atom. Saturated fats are solid at room temperature. They are generally more stable than unsaturated fats and go rancid less readily. Saturated fats are found in animal fats and tropical oils such as palm and coconut oils, and can also be overproduced in the body from the overeating of carbohydrates. (Hmm, interesting right?)

Butter	Cream (dairy)	Nutmeg Oil
Cheese	Fat	Shea nut oil
Ghee	Eggs	Sour Cream
Coconut oil		

Fats: Two types of unsaturated fats are: monounsaturated and polyunsaturated. Both are unstable at room temperature and are extremely sensitive to interaction with light, heat, and oxygen.

Monounsaturated Fats: Monounsaturated fats have a kink or bend at the position of the double bond and therefore do not pack together as easily as saturated fats, so they tend to be liquid at room temperature. They do not readily go rancid and are therefore able to withstand some cooking, but only at very low temperatures.

Almond oil	Grape-seed oil	Olive oil
Apricot Kernel oil	Hazelnut oil	Peanut oil
Avocado oil	Mustard oil	Rice oil
Canola oil (non-GMO)	Oat oil	

Polyunsaturated Fats: These oils are extremely susceptible to heat, light, and oxygen and should absolutely not be used for cooking. The most common types of polyunsaturated fats found in our diets are unsaturated linoleic acid, with two double bonds missing, known as "omega-6," and triple unsaturated linoleic, with three double bonds missing, known as "omega-3."

These oils are essential parts of our diet and must be treated with care.

Never heat these types of oil.

Herring oil	Salmon oil	Sesame seed oil
Wheat germ oil	Flaxseed oil	

Fats to Avoid

Trans-fats: A trans-fat might start out as a polyunsaturated oil, but due to its processing and exposure to high heat, the natural configuration known as "cis," with the molecules on the same side of the double bond, flips and becomes an unnatural "trans" formation. "Trans" means the hydrogen atoms are on opposite sides of the double bond. The human body does not contain the enzymes necessary to fully metabolize the trans fat into energy. When you eat trans-fatty acids, you end up with debris that clogs your cells and contributes to metabolic aging.

Be aware of the health myths out there regarding choices of oils. Many fast-food chains have switched from saturated oils to polyunsaturated oils, claiming them to be a better health choice. In fact, the polyunsaturated oils are extremely toxic when they are exposed to heat, light, and oxygen, and cause free radical damage in the body.

Hydrogenated Oils: It is important to be familiar with the terms "hydrogenated" and "partially hydrogenated." These oils are created when natural polyunsaturated oil has been altered by a chemical process that adds a hydrogen molecule to the fat molecule. This process is what changes an oil that was once liquid at room temperature to an oil that is solid at room temperature. This is how margarine is made. These types of oils, often found in items such as crackers, chips, and shortening, should be avoided. They are incredibly hard to digest or break down, and tend to accumulate in the body, which can contribute to elevated LDL cholesterol (bad cholesterol) and an array of other negative health issues.

A good rule of thumb:

Fats found in nature are healthy. Saturated, monounsaturated, and polyunsaturated fats are all natural fats and therefore are good for you, if treated with care.

Whole Carbohydrates

This group contains the three subgroups of fruit, whole grains, and starchy vegetables. Whole carbohydrates are highly recommended over refined carbohydrates because they are in their natural form and their nutrient density is much more accessible, and they also generally have a lower glycemic index. With essentially the same amount of calories, the food you eat when it is whole carbohydrate is way more potent, nourishing, and satisfying than when it's refined.

Avoid overeating refined carbohydrates in the form of high-glycemic breads, cereals, and pastas. Especially avoid refined carbohydrates that contain hydrogenated oils.

Interestingly, in the early years of the FDA, both public and political opinion agreed with this judgment. An article on the history of the FDA and its directors in *The Boulder Weekly,* a local newspaper, revealed the battle between refined and natural foods that was already raging almost a century ago:

The first director of the FDA was Dr. Wiley. Dr. Wiley was a vigilant and tireless crusader for the protection of the national health, foe of all adulterators of natural foods and makers of phony medicines. One of his first acts was to seize an imported shipment of refined and bleached white flour crossing interstate lines. He declared it an adulterated food, unfit for human consumption, and had all kinds of lab tests to prove it. He won in federal court and the case went all the way to the Supreme Court [which] ruled that, indeed, white flour was illegal. The very first shipment was sent back to China, as unfit for human consumption.

Very, Very Veggie

The United States Department of Agriculture (USDA) recommends we eat 7 to 13 servings of fruits and vegetables every day. But if you're like most people, you don't eat enough fruits or vegetables or a great enough variety of them. And those fruits and vegetables that you do eat tend to be over processed, overcooked, or too far removed from the field. It is important to consume as many organic vegetables as possible, as this is the best way to avoid consuming pesticides and chemical fertilizers. Organic vegetables are much higher in minerals due to the way organic farming rotates crops and naturally fertilizes soil. Our standard non-organic farms deplete the soil of the most vital nutrients, leaving our produce mineral-deficient. This is the leading cause of mineral deficiency in our society today—a major contributor to the lack of nourishment many people experience. The amount of pesticides and fertilizers ultimately depletes the food of its natural nutrients, leaving them weak and full of a wide assortment of toxins. As concerned, environmentally aware citizens, let's do our part for Mother Earth and support organic farming. Eat your greens, and try to do it locally if possible!

Water

Medical experts across the globe have accepted many health benefits of water. It is the most abundant compound present on this planet. All living forms require water in some way or another for their metabolic activities. We have gotten further and further away from the purity of drinking straight water with the increase in consumption of soda, juice, and other store-bought beverages. Increasing your water consumption to about ½ your body weight in ounces per day is what I encourage clients to strive for in both day-to-day life and during cleanse programs. Due to the major toxicity found in tap water, including traces of heavy metals, medications such as Prozac and birth control pills, and many other toxic chemicals, please drink purified water if at all possible.

Fact: The human body maintains a pH range of 7.35-7.45 for proper physiological processes. An acidic shift may lead to sickness, inflammation, and an inability to assimilate vitamins and minerals. Thus, your pH level should be above 7, which is favorable to your body's oxygen uptake, higher energy levels, and better immune response to diseases. This is more attainable by consuming appropriate amounts of purified water for your body.

Metabolism: Water is the carrier of oxygen, nutrients, and hormones to the various parts of our body, and it also provides a medium for the removal of toxins, dead cells, waste material, etc. Therefore it's a key component for a healthy metabolism. The proteins and enzymes involved in various fundamental processes also require water for effective detoxification and liver metabolism.

Cleansing

One of the only ways to truly purify your body of some of these common toxins is through cleansing. There are many ways to cleanse the body. Some cleanses are quite simple while others are more technical and complex. Starting with a whole food-based cleanse, and moving towards something based on more in-depth scientific research will give you a good idea of what feels right for you and your body!

According to *The New American Diet,* "Obesogens are chemicals that disrupt the function of our hormonal system, leading to weight gain and many of the diseases that curse the American populace. They enter our bodies from a variety of sources—everything from compounds found in processed soy products, from artificial hormones fed to our animals, from plastic pollutants in some food packaging, from chemicals added to processed foods, to pesticides sprayed on our produce. They act in a variety of ways— from mimicking human hormones such as estrogen, to blocking the action of other hormones such as testosterone, and, in some cases, altering the functions of our genes and essentially programming us to gain weight."

Increased trace mineral intake, enzyme-rich protein, and deep cellular nourishment combined with whole food and seasonal meals equals my ultimate cleanse program. When I follow this program, I see many long-term phenomenal health benefits, and I feel better than ever on every level, from sleep patterns to digestion to energy!

Although it is often challenging to make this shift away from the normal day-to-day snack foods and quick meals comprised mostly of processed foods and refined carbohydrates, the results are well worth the effort. Our bodies will work and feel so much better, while more effectively providing the energy and vitality we need to thrive. Many of our chronic health issues will self-resolve as a result, and we will have the opportunity to re-evaluate what feeling great looks and feels like. This is a gift that will always be with us as we age gracefully, feeling our best and enjoying life to the fullest. Our health is everything! The most important take-home practices here are that we eat simple whole foods daily, cleanse regularly, and begin to reclaim our natural state of health.

MEET ANN

Ann lives in Fort Collins, Colorado. She is a manager at a family health center, and a child and family therapist. When she was introduced to the cleansing process shortly after she moved to Colorado in 2006, she noticed she was becoming more health-conscious in Colorado than in her previous life in the Midwest. "Thank goodness cleansing became more trendy!" she says. Ann had hypoglycemia and migraines, and just was not feeling good at all. She felt really overweight, sluggish, and low energy. Her career of the past 18 years was incredibly stressful. Weight crept on, and her activity level crept lower, until just walking around was tough and tired her out. Ann says: "I didn't want to spend the rest of my life feeling bad. It was getting harder and harder to feel good!"

Ann completed my 11-day cleanse program focusing on detoxing the cells and resetting the metabolism. She then continued on with a rigorous maintenance program of regular cleansing and whole food eating. Ann has lost 25 pounds in 3 months. Last time she measured inches, she was down a total of 22 over her whole body, 3 around her waist. She feels that the 11-day cleanse program was the ticket! (More info on cleansing at www.HealthWise-Woman.com/foodandfreedom.) ~

"Cleansing has reset my system to not crave starch and sweets. Got me off the same old cycle of doing something and then feeling guilty. I am not succumbing to the emotional roller coaster associated with emotional eating.

I realized how much energy had been wasted in this beating up cycle. The results were so fast. I lost 8 pounds in 11 days. Stabilizing my blood sugar really helps with my migraines. With other diets I feel so deprived, and it is unsustainable, but the cleanse process feels do-able and balanced, and I feel it is achievable."

Ann plans on regular cleansing on an ongoing basis. She feels physically better, and realizes "detoxing" is real, and she really has achieved something. She is now always checking in and looking at how to feel more and more in tune with herself.

"Other diets are focusing on the wrong thing . . . CALORIES . . . and it does not work at all! I can eat so much less than I thought of nutrient-dense food and feel fantastic.

The 11-day cleanse program I completed the first time slowed me down enough to think about what I was eating. Eating whole foods and watching how much better I felt was huge. I have seriously been poisoning myself for years. Something clicked and I just didn't want to do it anymore!!! Even my little indulgences are much more manageable, much smaller, and not as bad for me. Cleansing has changed what tastes good to me in the big picture. All the support I received from my coaches was REALLY helpful."

There is plenty more information about seasonal cleanse programs on the Health Wise website at www. HealthWise-Woman.com/foodandfreedom. ♀

KEY #2: USE HIGH-QUALITY SUPPLEMENTS

In this day and age, we have so many choices for nutritional supplementation, but hardly any informative direction. From a holistic medicine approach, each individual, and his or her whole history and health status, are what determines appropriate supplementation including such elements as dosage, quality control, and individual response.

A big common question seems to be: Do I need to supplement??? I am a firm believer in supplementation. Supplements are like these little nuggets of information that educate our cells about how to work, heal, and run our bodies in the most effective way. Sometimes they get a bad rap in various media, and YES, the quality DOES matter, but if you are selective, informed, and wise about your supplement intake and quality, you will see both long-term benefits and short-term accelerated healing. So YES, most of us need supplements! They boost our energy, send high-powered antioxidants through our bodies, and provide balanced nutrition and high-powered super fuel we can almost always use to improve our health, either preventatively or to treat our health issues.

It is important to note that each individual may need a customized approach to supplementation. But most of us benefit from a basic program that consists of a multivitamin and EFAs (essential fatty acids). Treating metabolic issues, osteoporosis, gut dysbiosis, depression or mood imbalances, menopausal symptoms, skin issues, and heart disease, just to name a few, requires specific clinical doses of particular supplements based on personal health history. Once again, remember that basic complete nourishment of the cells can take care of a large portion of healing. When the cells are fully nourished, purified, and functioning optimally, they can then do their job to keep you healthy.

Why do we use supplements?

Supplements, at the most basic level, are designed to totally nourish the cells. When the cells are nourished fully they can maintain, heal, and vitalize the body, meeting all its needs for total health. Supplements bridge the gap that most of us have when it comes to nutrition due to the lack of minerals and nutrients in the soil and the resultant lack of vitality in our current commercial foods (even the high-quality ones).

It is also important to recognize the ways in which our population, as a whole, is deficient. These are the reasons why certain nutritional supplements will benefit most people today. The way our foods are grown and prepared these days leaves people depleted in many ways. Here it is important to see where some specific supplementation is supportive for the majority of the population. I recently read a study showing that the nutrient density of an orange in the early 1900s was eight times more potent in vitamins and minerals than an orange is today, especially in the trace mineral department. Wow! That means you would need to eat eight oranges today to benefit your body the way one orange would have 100 years ago!

Even the American Medical Association reversed its stance in the past decade, from saying no one needed supplements, to now advocating that all adults take supplements.

Remember, taking supplements is not an excuse to eat poorly. You still need to eat as well as you can—supplements won't single-handedly restore your health from the effects of a imbalanced unhealthy diet.

Foundational Supplements

Most nutritional supplements have multidimensional functions in the body. Some examples of these supplements are high-quality multivitamins, B vitamins, omega-3 fatty acids, and antioxidants.

Omega-3's

Studies show the effects of fish oil (a common omega-3) being highly supportive for the average person. Because our Western diet is low in omega-3's relative to other types of oils such as omega-6's and omega-9's, it is important to rebalance the ratio. Supplementation with omega-3 oils is highly beneficial for many reasons. Omega-3 fatty acids are important in the structure of cell membranes, and in overall cellular health. Omega-3 fatty acids help maintain normal functioning of the various hormonal systems and the immune system. Omega-3 fats are the structural material from which many important hormones are made such as vitamin D, DHEA, progesterone, testosterone, estradiol, and cortisol. Individuals struggling with mood imbalances often benefit from the addition of good quality supplements into their program. The

American Journal of Clinical Nutrition published a study in August 2000 confirming that the effects of a fish oil concentrate in postmenopausal women decreased the risk for cardiovascular disease by lowering LDL cholesterol levels. The study confirmed a reduced risk of twenty-seven percent. Therefore, for those who commonly face insulin resistance and hypothyroidism, it is clear that they will benefit from a high-quality omega-3 supplement. There are a couple of potent plant-based omega-3 supplements if that is your preference. Flax oil and chia seeds are both good options if you are a vegetarian or are allergic to fish. Both are high in omega-3's.

Antioxidants

Eating an antioxidant-rich diet is important for many aspects of health. It is virtually impossible to get the optimal amount of antioxidants through food alone. Some of the most common antioxidants are vitamin E, vitamin C, lipoic acid, and coenzyme Q10. These specific antioxidants are unique because of their synergistic qualities when taken together. Each of them works independently in the body in different ways, but they also work together, recycling each other and greatly enhancing one another's work. As a result these antioxidants are highly effective in slowing down the aging process and boosting the body's ability to fight disease.

Many nutritional companies make a combination supplement for a complete antioxidant formula. Antioxidants work with the body to promote overall health, balancing the hormones and keeping the organ systems of the body functioning at their optimal potential while keeping the cells protected in a favorable environment.

Note: Fermented foods such as kimchi, miso, kefir, and sauerkraut have increased antioxidant and probiotic properties as a result of the fermentation process. In many cultures they are used to increase the nutrient density of many meals.

Most people today could use therapeutic refinement of their diets through food and nutritional supplementation. It is difficult to obtain all of our nutritional requirements in our food alone in this day and age. Look for high-quality, high-grade, natural supplements with no additives or preservatives. Pharmaceutical grade supplements are guaranteed to be composed of the purest ingredients, and have the highest absorbability and most potent combinations.

The Importance of Quality Control

Because poor manufacturing can destroy great science, one must thoroughly research and verify the quality of supplements before beginning use. For example, to ensure that the formulas developed in high-quality company laboratories are produced consistently, the manufacturing processes should be consistent for every batch of supplement product. Every dietary supplement produced by a pharmaceutical grade company carries a potency guarantee, which ensures that what is stated on the label is actually contained in the product. Thus, pharmaceutical grade supplements are the safest—and most effective—option.

Current Regulations

The Federal Drug Administration has not finalized Good Manufacturing Practice (GMP) for dietary supplements, as they are theoretically required to do under the Dietary Supplement Health and Education Act. Rather, Congress has stated, as a provision, that dietary supplement GMP should be modeled after food regulations. Because of this statement, many supplement manufacturers have chosen to follow the GMP for foods. Others, however, voluntarily follow GMP for pharmaceuticals as the basis for their quality assurance program in the manufacturing of all of their products, meaning these companies treat the manufacture of nutritional supplements with the same care and consistency with which pharmaceutical companies treat the manufacture of theirs.

The NutriSearch *Comparative Guide to Nutritional Supplements* by Lyle MacWilliam gives a very thorough analysis of 1500 supplement companies in North America. It is a very useful resource when selecting a supplement to take. Be sure to purchase the most recent edition (the 4th edition, at the time of this printing). You can find links and more information about the *Comparative Guide* on the Health Wise website. www. HealthWise-Woman.com/foodandfreedom. ♀

Overall, caring for our health has gone from something that was once relatively simple and easy to something that requires a high degree of attention, education, and diligence. We have to step outside of the mainstream ways and rebalance our systems by maybe doing things a little differently than they used to be done. The simplicity of just "eating" has changed, as have the processes that produce most mainstream foods. It is our job to remember how the ways of respecting the land, eating pure whole foods, and using a natural, simple approach to ingredients can not only support our own health but also have a large ripple effect on the health of our planet.

KEY # 3: LEARN YOUR METABOLIC TYPE

Metabolism Defined

Metabolism is generally defined as the amount of energy a person's body burns. However, burning energy is only a small fraction of what your metabolism does. Metabolism is comprised of the combined effects of a variety of biochemical processes that continually occur in your body to help it function, making it possible for you to think, digest food, move, and perform all the functions of a living, breathing being. Some of these functions include: bone and tissue regeneration, elimination, fertility, functions of the internal organs, mood, vision, hormone production, heart function, sleeping, and even talking.

Your metabolism is essentially the power behind your entire system as a whole—the way your body processes all the input and transforms it into all the output. The interesting thing is that we all experience metabolism differently.

What works for one person may not work for another. "One woman's medicine is another's poison." Learning how your body runs at this very foundational level is something that will guide you in understanding yourself better, and also in learning what your particular body requires for optimal health and energy.

Metabolic Type ® Testing

Metabolic Type® testing is a profound tool based on scientific testing that informs us about how we metabolize our foods. Metabolic type® testing will help determine the ratio of protein, carbohydrates, and fats that are best for you. Based on the results, it will be easier to determine how you should be eating to stay healthy, nourished, and at your ideal body composition. The two ways to determine your Metabolic Type® are through a blood test or through a comprehensive online questionnaire. With this type of testing specific to the individual, a deeper understanding of how your body metabolizes food becomes apparent. As with any practice, this testing works better for some than for others. But for many people, Metabolic Type® testing provides another key to fostering a more balanced and nourished you.

There are nine metabolic types in the system I use, which comes from Dr. William Wolcott, who wrote *The Metabolic Typing Diet.* This system incorporates the autonomic nervous system, the cellular oxidation system, and the endocrine system of an individual. The necessary information can be generated via an online questionnaire. (www.HealthWise-Woman.com/ foodandfreedom). ♀

Once you establish how your body is metabolizing energy and how you can find the perfect balance of protein: fat: carbohydrate, you are then able to keep your metabolism at its best, feeling more energized and better than ever. Creating a customized plan to provide the perfect balance for your cells makes a huge difference in how you feel, how you age, and how much energy you have, and even in the release of excess body weight!

MEET JULIA

Julia is a 36-year-old woman who lives in Denver, Colorado. I met her at a yoga studio where I was guest speaking. She enjoys running, yoga, Pilates, tennis, and hanging out with her dog.

Julia works in the sports community. We started working together in the fall because Julia really wanted to prevent the Seasonal Affective Disorder (SAD) that usually hit her hard around January and February.

Julia shares: "With seasonal affective disorder I was sleeping 14 hours per night, putting on 10 to 12 pounds per winter, and waking up daily feeling like I wanted to cry. Working with the Metabolic Type® diet, adding in high-quality supplements, everything changed, my energy level improved in a positive way in the winter months. I had no weight gain, no carbohydrate cravings, no Homer Simpson living inside of me! JOY."

Julia has made a shift to eating more protein (she turned out to be a fast-oxidizer on her Metabolic Type® Test) at every single meal, avoiding high-glycemic carbohydrates, and taking regular supplements, including omega-3's, a high-potency multivitamin, vitamin D3, and tryptophan.

"If I do eat carbohydrates I am careful they are whole and low glycemic," she says.

Julia's long-term plan is to continue to keep the high-glycemic foods out and find new, exciting ways to keep protein intake up:

"The raw whey-protein shakes, buffalo meat, organic sausage, and eggs combined with a good amount of veggies are a key to success for me! This can truly let me focus on the rest of my life. Now I can focus on the stuff that is fun and positive, and relax more."

It feels awesome to be at an optimal weight, but in reality the energy and strength that come with proper health is a much bigger bonus."

Once we receive the guidance, the shift can happen. Before working with the Metabolic Type® test, Julia did not totally understand what she needed, even despite her efforts and self-taught information. A lot of effort and commitment was needed to get there, but now things are working well for her, so it was well worth it. As Julia says, "Now, even if I lose balance, I know how to bring myself back."

KEY #4: PRACTICE INTUITIVE EATING

Once we understand the first three keys—eating a whole-food diet, using high-quality supplementation, and learning your Metabolic Type® —we can move ahead to the practice of *intuitive eating*. Without the solid foundation we have just covered, we would be asking our intuition to reach outside of our current map of inner knowledge and experience.

Intuitive eating is the ability to listen inward and tune into the body's own instinctual cues and mechanisms, which are naturally in place for our own health and well-being. We see this so clearly in the animal world. In fact, as Michael Pollan, food and food politics expert, states: "We are the only species on the planet who have lost the ability to know what we need to eat." It is possible to reconnect to the ability to read ourselves, and our needs in a new intuitive and health-wise way. It does take some letting go, some self-study, some purification, but rest assured, with practice, it is totally possible.

Intuitive eating becomes a practice that is strengthened over time with more exposure to what works and what doesn't work. Here are some ideas to consider when you are re-defining your relationship with food, freedom, and your highest good.

Eating when you are hungry: This may sound so simple, yet so many of us struggle with our relationship to hunger. We often think we are hungry, but really our minds are hungry. Sitting and watching our hunger for a moment before we act on it is such a great practice to deepen into what is really happening. Of course sometimes we are truly hungry, but sometimes we are actually bored, emotionally riled up, or even feeling self-destructive.

Your mind and your body have completely different needs, but your mind has control of your body. Your body has needs that you cannot avoid; you have to fulfill the need for food, the need for water, shelter, sleep, and sex. All those needs are completely normal, and easy to satisfy. The problem is that the mind says, "these are MY needs." In the mind we create a whole picture in the bubble of illusion, and the mind takes responsibility for everything. The mind thinks it has the need for food, for water, for shelter, for clothing, and for sex. But the mind has no needs at all, no physical needs that is. The mind does not need oxygen, doesn't need water, and doesn't need sex at all. How do we know this is true? When you need food, you eat, and the body is completely satisfied, but your mind still thinks it needs food. You keep eating and eating and eating, and you cannot satisfy your mind with food, because that need is not real. When the need is in the mind, you cannot satisfy the need. To free ourselves from this cycle of suffering, we need to separate the needs we experience into two categories:

1. *The needs of the body.*
2. *The needs of the mind.*

The mind easily confuses the body with its own needs simply because the mind needs to know "What am I?" The affinity between the mind and the body is so close that the mind can easily believe "I am the body" . . . This is our work! You take away what is not you, until in the end the only thing that remains is what you really are. It's a long process of the mind finding its own identity. In the process, you let go of the personal story, what makes you feel safe, until finally you understand what you really are.

— *Don Miguel Ruiz, The Mastery of Love*

Knowing the signs

- Be alert for the signs of true physical hunger, such as a physical sensation in the stomach, growling, contracting, and gnawing.

- Watch for a drop in your energy, vitality, and blood sugar. Take a few moments to get to know your hunger. Watch, witness without acting on it for a while, until you become clear that it is physical hunger. Let it have a voice and time to be heard. I always tell my clients to wait, listen, and see what comes.

- Be patient with yourself. Food is a way we often self-soothe, check out, and even cover up fearful emotions or strong feelings. Skillful listening to these cues can help you understand what you are really needing in order to feel nurtured and taken care of.

What are you hungry for?

Once you identify whether or not you are truly physically hungry, can you identify what it is you are hungry for? This is a skill that is great to hone as you practice intuitive eating. Sometimes you may need protein, or even more fat in your diet. Sometimes you may crave something with key nutrients that your body needs after a long workout or stressful day. Maybe you find you are craving red meat or heavier proteins right before your monthly period. All of this information is key for you to be aware of to help you refine your intuition and pay attention to the deeper needs for your body temple to thrive.

Stop eating when you are full.

When we eat a diet that is closer to nature and more balanced to our metabolic type, it helps satiate us and we get a clearer signal when it's time to stop eating. Interestingly enough, foods that are high in sugar, refined carbohydrates, and processed ingredients have a slower reaction time, and don't give us the cues from our brains to our stomachs to stop eating in time. We don't recognize that we are full until it is too late. Therefore, these foods are often the ones we overeat! With this said it is obvious that intuitive eating is simply harder to do when we eat a diet high in processed and refined foods. No wonder so many of us struggle. Learning to stop overeating comes much more easily when we purify our diets and eat more simply! Get off the sugar train and things will shift.

These are tools that are so simple in concept, but quite challenging in practice. Trusting the process is part of the journey. Your body is absolutely designed to tell you what it needs. In modern society, where we are eating more processed foods that are infused with many additives, preservatives, and strong flavors such as salt, sugar, and refined oils, our inherent wisdom can be blocked. Our map of intuition can be limited. With practice we begin to be able to separate intuition from habits and emotional cravings, and to allow our nutritional needs to be met in a holistic, body-wise experience.

KEY # 5: CONSCIOUS EATING

This next key really brings it all together for me. As a yogini I resonate with the idea of making our eating experience a spiritually or mindfully based one—bringing awareness to how we eat, where we eat, and what we are doing when we are eating. In our modern culture we are often bombarded by constant rushing, high stress, and a fast-paced lifestyle, all of which prevents many of us from slowing down enough to prepare and enjoy our food. We often eat on the run, in our cars, standing up over the sink, or even making the occasional drive through the fast-food joint for the sake of convenience. The practice of conscious eating is one that many complain they don't have time for, yet the yearning for health, happiness, and feeling good in our bodies is what many of us strive for.

Just as we learn to find the mindfulness in the "chop wood, carry water" approach to day-to-day life, we can practice taking the time to slow down, finding gratitude for our food, breathing mindfully, and staying present as we eat. We are then prepared to listen inward to the experience of eating, and find satiation from our food in a whole new way. For example, did you know that eating in a calm space puts the parasympathetic (calming) side of your nervous system in action, and you are actually able to absorb the nutrients from your food much more effectively?

Here are some great tips for mindful eating:

1. **Create mealtime in a calm space, free from distractions and stress:** Avoid eating around over stimulating technology or stressful situations and conversations. Eating in a peaceful setting is self-nourishment as a meditation or mindfulness practice.

2. **Feng-shui your kitchen:** You may need to clean out your cupboards and set up your kitchen in a way that inspires you, and that also removes the unhealthy foods that are too tempting to be around! Bri Maya Tiwari speaks of this often in her book, *The Path of Practice*. The way we relate to our kitchen space, food choices, and how we prepare our food, all has a huge impact on how our body receives food, nourishment, and overall health.

3. **Slow Food:** Slow down and create sacred space by listening to peaceful music, lighting a candle, setting the table, setting out flowers, and making mealtime a time to unwind, rest, and nourish yourself. Eating slowly

is a monumental shift for our bodies and our bodily cues. Chew your food, taste your food, and you will be blown away by how much your experience can shift.

KEY # 6: FOOD AS PLEASURE AND CELEBRATION

Most of us have experienced, at a special event, gathering or party, the joy found in eating and sharing good food with others. Food brings people together in pleasure, with its delicious accents to the senses, giving us the opportunity to collectively experience the flavors, the smells, and the textures. Food adds so much beauty to a lifestyle of health, community, and celebration. When we eat with pleasure, mindfulness, and balance, we actually activate the good hormones in the body—the ones that increase our metabolisms and literally get us into the fat-burning zone—and decrease those stress hormones that do us no favors for weight gain or self-control. This allows us to slow down and be mindful. It is such good news that more pleasure with food equals more lean body mass, more balanced hormones, greater absorption, and more soul nourishment. This science-based information is enough to remind us to celebrate food, not just for the fun of it, but also for the health of it.

What we have covered up to this point is simply good balanced eating. Now this new component of eating as celebration is designed to open us to more joy and pleasure than we could imagine—joy and pleasure that are truly sustainable. If we apply all of the keys we spoke of earlier, and then infuse our eating with creativity, inspiration, and community, the enjoyment can be immeasurable. The good news is this expansion into more enjoyment with food will permeate other areas of our lives.

Food For Thought

Although food can feel like an area of challenge for many, coming home to a healthy daily practice around it is absolutely a form self-love ("ahimsa") and self-care. We are inherently designed to use our intuition and instincts and we need to remember what it means to nourish ourselves on all levels, to live close to nature, and to open to more and more joy in our experience of food.

The practice of implementing these six keys will offer a journey back home to our own truth, connection, and the inner freedom that we so deserve in our relationship to our health, to our food, and to our overall life experience. This primary source of nourishment we all have in common, food, is complex yet profound. This is a journey to higher consciousness—to deeper levels of knowing our selves and our bodies, while empowering ourselves through one of our most primary relationships to date: our relationship with food. This is fundamental healing that can awaken our sense of well being and remind us that our inherent wholeness is untouchable. The ahimsa we can turn inward and live within ourselves becomes our inner guide for all aspects of life.

HOME PRACTICE

1.   *Write a food journal for 1 week and begin to watch the patterns in your relationship with food, including emotional cravings, energy, and sleep quality. (Food journal downloadable templates available at www.HealthWise-Woman.com/foodandfreedom)* ♀

2.   *Create 3 fantastic breakfast ideas for yourself. (Visit the website:* HealthWise-Woman.com/foodandfreedom *for some amazing recipes and power smoothie ideas.) Use a variety of power smoothies for on-the-go mornings.*

3.   *Commit to eating breakfast like a queen for 1 month (make sure it includes some kind of healthy protein). This practice will balance and reset your metabolism drastically and you will begin to clearly see any emotional eating patterns in a different light.*

4.   *Find a buddy to cleanse with. Visit the website* (HealthWise-Woman.com/foodandfreedom) *to find out about upcoming facilitated cleanse programs.* ♀

Bonus Practice:

BONUS Documents on www.HealthWise-Woman.com/ foodandfreedom ♀

- *Recommended Foods List*

- *Glycemic Index Chart*

- *Learn your Metabolic Type*

6 Keys to Food and Freedom Overview

Key #1: Simplify-Purify: *Eat a whole food, local, organic diet, and cleanse your body seasonally.*

Key #2: Use High-Quality Supplements: *Quality, purity, and potency matter.*

Key #3: Self-Study: *Learn your metabolic type and how to take care of your individual needs down to a metabolic level.*

Key #4: Practice Intuitive Eating: *Listen to what your body wants and needs.*

Key #5: Conscious Eating: *Food as a mindfulness practice.*

Key #6: Celebrating Food: *Expanding into joy, creativity, and pleasure with food. Celebrate and connect with others to enhance the senses, community, and celebration.*

SECRET #3

Flip your Script

Change your thoughts if you wish to change your circumstances. Since you alone are responsible for your thoughts, only you can change them. Each thought creates according to its own nature . . .

—Paramahansa Yogananda

One of the most important aspects of creating health in every area of life is working with the ever-present internal dialogue, our very own thoughts. The way we talk to ourselves all day long is constantly impacting our internal experience and quality of life, and also directly affecting the external experience we are creating for ourselves in the world. What we focus on gets stronger, so if we find ourselves focusing on the negative, or strengthening our negative internal dialogue and thought patterns, we may actually be manifesting exactly what we don't want in our lives. We all know how it feels to "beat ourselves up" versus "talk ourselves up" in our own heads. One of the most significant factors in our overall daily health is our way of thinking. This is often the crux, as this area is one place we commonly feel out of control, with the impression that our thoughts run crazy and have a mind of their own. The truth is, with practice, we can begin to reclaim control of our internal script, and cleanse our minds. Yes, you do have the ability to pull the reins in on your monkey mind, and create an internal dialogue that will not only better serve you but will also be much more pleasant to listen to!

Our internal dialogue, combined with our paradigms of belief, is the filter through which we see the world. It is the perspective we have about ourselves that can so greatly promote and attract our vision, and our health, or greatly sabotage it.

Many say a daily practice such as yoga or meditation will clear the lens through which we see the world. With practice it is possible to have a new experience with our thoughts and to actually flip our script from negative and unsupportive to positive and uplifting, which will really and truly begin to shift our lives from the inside out.

One of the most sacred and powerful laws of the universe, as seen in "The Secret" and written about in so many books and publications both ancient and modern, is how to use the "law of attraction" to benefit our overall experience. The internal dialogue is foundational to the law of attraction. According to the *law of attraction,* creating the life we desire begins with examining our internal dialogue and our deep-rooted belief systems. If we can begin to release the beliefs and thoughts that do not serve our highest good, and replace them with the highest vibration of thought aligned with our truth and our desire for a fulfilling life, then we can begin to create the healthy, hopeful, joyful existence that is our divine birthright. It just takes practice, repetition, and commitment...

EXAMINING OUR PARADIGMS OF BELIEF

Our paradigms of belief are the day-to-day belief systems that are ingrained in our beings, usually instilled in us from a young age. They are decisions that we have made throughout our lives for which we have then, both consciously and subconsciously, collected evidence to prove to be "true." They are the very lens, or perspective, through which we see the world.

The paradigm in which we operate is the sum of our beliefs, values, identity, expectations, attitudes, decisions, opinions, and thought patterns about ourselves, others, and life. To shape your future you have to be ready and able to transform your current paradigm into one that supports you and attracts the right energy to you for you to step into your fullest potential.

NEW PATHWAYS

Unfortunately, our existing internal dialogue is like an overused major highway in our brains, and to create a new experience, we have to literally create new roads in our neurotransmitter pathways. Just like any new road, in the beginning, this requires a fair amount of bushwhacking, maybe even getting lost, until the "deer trail" becomes a footpath and eventually a neighborhood drive.

As you begin the process of replacing old beliefs or dialogues with new ones, it is common to notice that all the evidence you have spent your whole life gathering to prove your current belief system is still in your file box. It will come up, it may scream loud and strong, and it may feel like the case it makes against these new, more affirming, thoughts will win hands down. Don't be fooled! The good news is, as you keep practicing the awareness that leads you to paying attention to these types of thoughts and beliefs, you are honing your skills and training your mind to think in a more favorable way for your future of mental health, positive thinking, and creating the life and health you want for yourself.

This type of practice impacts many, many aspects of your daily experience. If you spend just a few minutes a day listening to your internal dialogue, you may be truly shocked. Most of us wouldn't even talk to our own children, friends, or family, in the negative, shame-inducing, critical tones in which we often talk to ourselves. It is imperative to address our internal dialogue if we are wanting to live in happiness, radiance, and health.

WHO WROTE THE SCRIPT?

One of the exercises to deepen awareness around these ever-present internal dialogues is to examine who wrote the script. You may automatically think it was you, of course, but in actuality, with some inquiry into the deeper meanings and histories of these beliefs, you may find that there were certain influences that had a large part in the process.

Our families are obviously one of the central and most common sources of these beliefs, but surely this is not limited to just them. I often think of these dialogues as someone's voice getting inside my head, and I begin to personify them into different characters. This way I am separated from the voices, and I can choose to listen or take them on, or not, from a conscious place. You may find that some of the beliefs you received from your childhood truly serve you, but maybe a sibling, teacher, or friend at some point in your life has also negatively influenced the voices that keep playing over and over, leaving you feeling depleted, defeated, and ashamed. Yes?

Can you relate? Marc David, founder of the Institute for the Psychology of Eating, one of our country's foremost health gurus, and a good friend of mine, stated in a recent talk, "You are not one person, you are a crowd." I notice, for example, that my internal voices change according to stress, PMS, family dynamics, and especially fatigue. If I am exercising, living my purpose, and getting enough rest, I do better. The minute I put myself out of balance, surround myself with negative environments or people, or burn myself out, I tend to default to these old, and almost "lazier," thought pathways that actively sabotage my success.

The first step is to watch. Take some time each day to witness or listen from an objective place, as if you were sitting back and watching a dialogue on stage. Feel free to really characterize the different components to allow even more personification. This will start to unravel the voices into something that makes sense and can transform into a dialogue that truly supports you in your life more and more!

Somewhere in there is your true self, your higher self, the self that you want to be cultivating daily, and nurturing on a continual basis. Identifying this voice is really important. Once you are able to discern the voices that are sabotaging you and keeping you small, you can begin the work to shift them. The deep light, divinity, and truth of you speaks in a way that uplifts you. It doesn't sugarcoat, deny, or avoid your taking responsibility, but it is your truth and the truth of your purpose. It is your heart, your love, you at your deepest, most heartfelt core place. From this place we are able to be free and powerful, and live in our highest potential.

All the other work around health loses its value and its potency if this layer is not working. In truth, this is the core of the work. If you only ever strive to work on the external, the outer layers, you will always be struggling somewhat, because you'll only be treating the symptom, not the actual source of the problem. Emerging from this work is your true essence, your belief and trust in yourself, and your strength, beauty, and light. Nothing is more powerful than alignment on this level. It may feel hard, and some days even impossible, but the light and positive energy has such a powerful impact on us that its true strength tends to always find the way. Practice, and trust!

BEGINNING THE SHIFT

The first step in creating positive internal dialogue is to notice the patterns. Where and when do you see these patterns arise? How can you begin to shift these thought habits that have been there since you can remember? Here are a few tricks that can support you in higher awareness around internal dialogue:

1.   **Sleep**

On some deep visceral level, we all know how important sleep is, and yet somehow we tend to selectively forget. Sleep is probably the #1 ingredient for health. It is #1 because it seems that everything else deteriorates with out it. In my experience working with hundreds of women around health, food, psychology, body image, etc., let me tell you, everything falls apart when we are sleep deprived. Our food choices go downhill, we don't have the energy to exercise, and if you expect yourself to actually have a positive internal dialogue when you are exhausted, I wish you the best of luck, as it is tough. If you simply can't sleep due to small children, or challenging sleep patterns, you must go easy on yourself, and work on getting those zzz's in order as best you can.

We are all unique as to the exact amount of sleep we need to thrive, but with a little experimenting, best done on the weekends when you can really follow your own sleep rhythm, free of alarm clock, sleep aids, and, of course, judgment, you can get a pretty good idea of your needs.

With this baseline, simply do the math and see what time you would need to go to bed to get a good amount of sleep before your workday begins. Add in a bit of leeway to allow for hormones, big exercise days, and our natural rhythms of the month and season, and hopefully you can come up with a range that you can then infuse with intuition and wisdom. With that said, there are simply times when you have no control, for example when you are breastfeeding through the night, or your six-year-old has a cough, or you are under high amounts of stress.

Learn to honor the time of the month when everything changes hormonally as you approach menstruation and you may need to spend more time resting. These are times of deep surrender when we have to dig deep and know that it is temporary. When all else fails, just hop into that comfy bed!

Creating a healthy and positive daily sleep ritual is key. Many of us do not realize that we are using electronics and TV, and even engaging in stress-inducing activities, right before bed. If you can give yourself even twenty minutes to unwind, read, take a warm bath, meditate, or drink a quiet cup of herbal tea, you will notice your nervous system unwinding and your sleep coming more easily. Even drinking caffeine earlier in the day can create a tough transition from day to night!

Did you know that your body's own natural melatonin is at its best in the darkest light? Even a small nightlight, alarm clock, or quick trip to the bathroom when the light goes on can mess up the melatonin production and interrupt sleep more than you think. Many people do well with a sleep mask, or blinds that keep the light out. Be aware of anything bright or light in your room as it could be the culprit in sleep disruption.

Try to keep your room full of relaxing scents and sounds. Create a peaceful, non-cluttered environment that brings you solace. Create a sacred space where you feel glad to go for relaxation, deep rest, and cellular repair. This is a key to your health, rejuvenation, and mental experience. As I said earlier, everything works better when we are rested! Your thoughts alone have so much impact on your day-to-day health, so with a rested mind, you would be surprised how much more clean and clear your thoughts can become.

2.   Somatic Resourcing

Choosing a resource that brings familiar positive memories, sensations, and feelings is a helpful way to shift out of a negative thought pattern or stress pattern. A resource is usually an object, place, or person. A resource should resonate positively in the nervous system. You should connect with warm, calming, and relaxing feelings in relationship to this object, place, or person.

When we connect with our resource, we are actually engaging in a somatic process to tell our bodies that we are okay, safe, and centered.

Using a resourcing technique in the moment can ease the nervous system and remind us of the positive relationship we have with ourselves and with life. This can literally redirect the thought process from destructive to constructive, stressed to relaxed. Generally we can improve the experience in the moment and feel better.

Practice

Choose an object that brings you positive memories or feelings. This could be your grandmother's pendant, a ring you bought on a fun trip, a crystal a friend gave you for your birthday, or even a rock that caught your eye on your favorite hike. Keep this object with you, around your neck, on your finger, or in your pocket to remind your nervous system to unwind and to come back to positive internal dialogue and a relaxed, pleasant state.

I have a pendant that I bought on a beach vacation with my two closest friends. We all bought similar necklaces and then we held a ritual in the local waterfall, intending our highest purpose and truth to be embedded in our pendants. Years later, I still often wear this necklace and it remains a resource for me to remember this trip and the intentions I set during our ritual. This helps me stay centered, and improves my feeling in the moment. As negative thoughts arise, hold or stroke your resourcing object and know that this will give your body a positive message and support a shift in your thoughts.

Try doing this for 7 days and see how much you can shift yourself into a more positive state. Watch your internal dialogue improve and observe how your overall mood and feeling becomes more grounded in the moment.

Some great examples of resourcing objects:

A favorite key chain
Necklace or pendant
Ring
Hair clip
Clothing item such as scarf or shoes
Jewel or crystal in your pocket
Favorite rock, including a heart-shaped rock
Picture on your desk
Application on your phone (I love the singing bowl app on my iPhone)
Lip balm/gloss
Wallet photo

3. Journal Writing

For many people it's helpful to keep a tiny notebook or journal accessible throughout the day to jot down a note anytime you notice a negative thought or belief arise. At the end of each day, go back and revisit what you experienced and write a small summary. Tracking each day will be interesting depending on daily stresses, certain people or situations that come up, where you are in your menstrual cycle, etc. All of these factors can influence the patterns of self-talk. Playing the witness in your life, especially with your thoughts, can be even more effective and accessible when your pen hits your paper.

4.   **Celebrate Your Successes Daily**

Often we wait for the moments of perfection, celebration, or monumental successes to acknowledge our hard work, commitment, and success. Wouldn't it be nice to be acknowledged for the small things as well—to be rewarded for simply being effective in a meeting, making good choices with food, or being patient with your toddler? Practicing positive self-talk, and strengthening the "muscles" around doing so, works very well to help you develop the internal dialogue you desire. It may feel a bit like the "fake it 'til you make it" approach, but practicing something new has to start somewhere. Forming a new habit takes some repetition, and in the meantime, you get a pat on the back for the day-to-day stuff that does take some hard work to keep up with and is so often overlooked.

We are going to get to some daily meditation practices (in Secret # 5) through which you can incorporate another way to watch, witness, and learn from some of your most common thoughts, as well as discerning where you can upgrade them to more hopeful, positive, supportive ones.

PAUSING THE RECORDING

Often the internal dialogue seems like a broken record. We all know what that is like. Remembering that these internal conversations are literally just thoughts is going to help you begin to slow them down enough to really see what is going on in there.

Pausing the recording is just a way to acknowledge that you have the power to engage with some of your thoughts and choose to let others free. Byron Katie, well-known author and speaker, talks about how we all share similar thoughts, and they are recycling through the collective consciousness over and over. What is going on in your head is probably similar to what is going on in the head of the woman behind you in line at the grocery store, or the head of the woman next to you at your son's kindergarten play. The important practice is noticing which thoughts you choose to latch onto that end up making up your internal dialogue. So hang in there, be patient with yourself, and meet life where life meets you. This is not a rigid process, but one that is always transforming, growing, and getting better and better with more and more awareness.

"Don't believe everything you think."

This is one of my favorite axioms—so full of wisdom and meaning. It holds a lot of truth. I often remind myself of this throughout the day. Ask yourself, "Is this thought really true?" You may be surprised . . . often our thoughts are far from the truth.

We tend to spend a lot of time working on the effect and getting no results. Why not go right to the source?

Event + Response = Outcome

Jack Canfield, well-known creator of the *Chicken Soup for the Soul* books, talks about this equation in relationship to our day-to-day successes. We so often get caught up in the events, and we can spend years trying to change the events in our lives to create a different outcome, when in reality the power to change lies in the response! We do have control over our responses, and we can start to shift them by practicing with thought and internal dialogue. That is exactly where responses are born. Health and success do not always come easy, but even from a place of defeat (which we have all—even the great legends of our time—experienced) we can still work with our responses in a conscious, intentional way.

In reality the only components you DO have control over in your life are the way you think, the way you act, and the vision you hold for what it is you want. If you want health, vitality, and happiness, then start with the way you talk to yourself. If thought precedes feelings, and feelings precede action and results, let's get right to those thoughts and shift them so they can begin to shift our experience on the outside more quickly!

I just want to clarify that I myself am nowhere near done, complete or mastered on this secret. It is a real doozy, but I do work diligently on it every single day. I work on it during my morning practice, in my journaling, and in my moment-to-moment awareness. I am committed to improving and shifting my internal dialogue always. I am not expecting miracles, but I am practicing, and I do see changes, improvements, and positive results.

AFFIRMATIONS

Positive affirmations are the beginning of shifting all that you are working with around the cause of your dis-harmony on the inside, rather than the effect your thoughts are having on the outside. Create an affirmation from your higher self as a way to replace an old pattern and create a new pattern of internal dialogue. For example, if you notice yourself constantly saying: *"I am not good enough,"* flip it around to something like *"I can do anything, I am strong, capable, and successful."* If you notice something more like, *"Why do I always F$%#ck* up so much? I just can't get it right,"* try something like, *"I am doing a great job in my life, I take care of myself, I love myself, and I share that with the world."* The best one I have seen was from a woman in one of my groups who was feeling unhappy, and uninspired in her sex life, and she needed an uplift. She chose to affirm, *"I am confident and beautiful, and a hot piece of ass!"* She got a lot of support from the group on that one!

The most important thing about creating a positive affirmation is that it resonates with you completely. It speaks to your heart, and you can get totally inspired down to a cellular level when hearing it often. Affirmations will literally change something that is not working into something that is working. They will create that new footpath we spoke of earlier, and allow those new pathways to continually strengthen. Affirmations need to be strong and clear. They need to be traveled frequently, and the more emotion, faith, and determination behind them, the better they will work. Try to keep them in the first person, and in the positive voice.

If you notice you have many "lines" of negative internal dialogue that run through your head frequently, create a few affirmations to match each one. Substitute the affirmations that support you for the habitual thought patterns that impede you.

THE DANCE PARTY

One of the quickest, most fun, and most effective ways to shift thought patterns in the moment is to turn on your favorite dance song and begin to move! Sometimes our energy gets stuck, and all the affirmations, meditation, or inquiry can feel like the most boring and stagnant approach. That is a sign that it is time to move!!! Shifting your feeling tone is really accessible through dance, and even singing or chanting (more on this in Secret #5). Get your groove on . . . we ABSOLUTELY have a virtual dance party waiting for you on the Health Wise website: www.

HealthWise-Woman.com/internaldialogue ♀

On my women's retreats called Waves of Bliss, in Costa Rica, we have a tradition of regular daily spontaneous dance parties. They totally work. It takes the ladies a few days to warm up but once we get rolling nothing can stop us! I am telling you, give it a try. I have one client who called me recently to tell me that she finally got the courage up to have her own private dance party at home, and it felt great! She even got up enough confidence over time to invite her boyfriend in. They had a blast. There are some starter songs for dance parties on the Health Wise website—check it out, and maybe it will be just the medicine you need to upgrade your thoughts and shift your internal dialogue to something more positive!

LIVING YOUR SUCCESS QUEEN

Take some space to introduce your internal success queen (you know the one) to your internal self-saboteur (we all have one of those too!). Give them about 3 to 5 minutes to have a little chat. You can do this quietly in a meditative place. Let them have an introduction and conversation, and learn from each other. After the 3 to 5 minutes are complete, take a little journal time as well. Well, what did they have to say to each other? What did each of them look like, sound like, or dress like?

I always find this exercise to be very profound. I use it with my women's groups and we always have a good laugh at how each of these energies are personified in our heads. Making peace with, and understanding, the roles the success queen and self-saboteur play is very helpful as you move forward in creating the life you want to live.

When I did this the first time, it was so interesting. I was on a live conference call with my dear friend Liza Pascal, and she was leading a business- coaching group. I was resistant, and thought, "Oh, here we go again with yet another self-help exercise." Can you believe the skeptic that can come out? But I went through the exercise for literally 3 minutes and had a surprisingly profound experience. My success queen was so confident, savvy, well dressed, and smart. Totally empowered! My self-saboteur was such an immature, childlike persona that was basically having a tantrum, acting out, and being quite a nuisance. It was that moment when I realized, "Hey, this saboteur is a child! Why am I letting her stop me from being totally in my success?" My success queen and saboteur had an interesting conversation about life, and as it turned out the saboteur just needed a little comfort and was acting out of fear. Have you ever seen a child act out in fear, sabotaging your plan? That was me! The point is that something I originally resisted, and that really only took 3 minutes, made a huge impact on me, and I soon began using this exercise with my women's groups. You can follow my guided meditation on this exercise on our interactive website. www.HealthWise-Woman.com/internaldialogue ♀

MOVING FORWARD WITH CONFIDENCE

The overall goal in this chapter is to investigate your thoughts and thought patterns and how they serve you— or not—in your life! One of the most common habits of successful people in just about any area of life is their use of the powers of the mind and thought. As you have clarified and maybe even discovered your purpose in secret #1, now secret # 3 is one of the best areas to work on, as our thoughts are most often our biggest obstacle to personal success, health, and happiness. Internal dialogue is usually where we can see the biggest breakthroughs as we begin to pay attention and shift our ways of thinking and witnessing ourselves. SHINE on!

HOME PRACTICE

1.   *Take some time to witness your internal dialogue and write down the top 3 thoughts that you notice sabotaging you throughout the day. Rewrite them, and create some positive affirmations to use in their place. Keep the affirmations inspiring, heartfelt, and meaningful to you.*

2.   *Do the Success Queen and Self-Saboteur Meditation and write down your experience. Have fun with it and see what comes! Visit the Health Wise interactive website for a live Success Queen meditation.*

3.   *Dance party! Next time your find yourself in a funk which is often a result of one or more negative thoughts, pick your favorite tunes and dance, dance, dance! You will be surprised by how it affects your mood and energy. If you feel awkward, just give it a minute and keep on keeping on. It will shift.*

Join us!

Be sure to visit
www.HealthWise-Woman.com/internaldialogue
for support and further strategies. ♀

Secret #4

Embracing The Feminine

Appreciate the fullness of your feminine intelligence, which comes not just through your intellect, but also through your body's cycles. Your feelings are also part of your intuition.

—Christiane Northrup, M.D.

Finding our paths as empowered women in today's world involves patience, practice, and a deep commitment to the feminine principle. Many of us have experienced repression and confusion as we have strived to embrace our true feminine essence. Following a path of truth, authenticity, and full embodiment of our sacred feminine helps us find our full radiance and health.

As a child I spent many years living the life of a tomboy. I wanted to be strong, tough, and athletic. All of these qualities were considered more stereotypically masculine, and therefore I wanted to be more masculine, hanging with the boys and honing my physical skills. I was a competitive athlete, and was terribly afraid of the oncoming changes in my body that would make me unmistakably a woman. I liked hanging out with other girls like me, but more so, with boys, to whom I could relate more readily. I still carry a seed of these qualities within me now, but each time I went through a rite of passage as a woman—menstruation (which happened quite late for me), pregnancy, and childbirth—I had to let go and step more and more into my true femininity, often with resistance and a feeling of discomfort. I gradually learned to put my shame and struggle aside, and open more to my inner guidance, trusting more, and really embracing myself as a woman.

It was challenging and surprising, and felt totally foreign at times, but with more support, and with a sense of delight in the true beauty and strength that do exist in the feminine, I learned to open more gracefully to myself.

I remember challenging the sixth-grade boys to arm wrestling matches and beating them every time. I also remember making the school record for the flexed arm hang, and feeling on top of the world—this was the type of recognition I was looking for. The qualities of diligence and determination that I developed in my quest for athletic prowess did turn out to serve me in many, many ways in my life, but now I often contemplate: what was it about being strong and tough that was so important to me? We all need to have our own way of expressing our feminine in the world. For some it is about equality, and for some it is about finding a balance in the subtle biology between masculine and feminine, stepping more into our strength. For me it was about softening, and learning to accept the fullness of the feminine within me, without running away and hiding from its glory.

In our culture it is challenging to find the power and strength in the feminine when living in such a masculine-dominated society. It has taken me a great deal of inner investigation and maturity to shift my own thinking and feel the empowerment inherent in the feminine, but once I began to connect with it, it blew my mind!

As we look back through the ages, we see how the feminine was revered, worshipped, and looked to for intuition, guidance, and wisdom. She was the goddess who many prayed to for abundance, prosperity, and fertility. She was the safe place where one could find nurturing, listening, and understanding. It is our collective task to reclaim this lost part of ourselves. It is time to find a balance, both globally and individually. It is our obligation to womanhood as a whole to remember the ways in which we can fully command the feminine in all its forms. It is our calling to trust that our beauty and power rest in the re-creation of the divine feminine for the modern, empowered woman—a woman who can own a business, work in corporate America, or manage the family finances, all from the seat of the feminine. This is the new, emerging paradigm. A woman who feels at home in her feminine beauty, alive in her motherhood (whether literal or energetic), and still able to live her passion and purpose in the world is finally being reborn on a larger scale. In the last 100 years we have successfully carried out many obligations, careers, and everyday responsibilities but, without the sacred feminine there to hold us as we unveil our power and purpose in the world, many of us have sacrificed our wholeness—the unification of our spiritual intuition and our practical approach to the day-to-day.

The divine feminine is the connection between spirit and matter, between intuition and finances, between unconditional love and wisdom.

Each of the three main life cycles that we go through as women (menstruation, childbirth, and menopause) signifies a different rite of passage, a different claim to our femininity, and even a different level of evolution within the divine feminine, both internally and externally. As we weave our sexuality, self-love, and self-expression into our lives, we develop a rich and colorful experience of life that is always changing and always teaching us.

We are being called to listen.

As we explore each of these three very significant times and passageways, we can find ways to heal our past experiences, as well as to create an authentic feminine expression as we move ahead into harmony within and without, for our own futures and for the futures of those who learn from us. Therefore these passageways are a vehicle to dive deeper, listen more, heal the past, and learn that our femininity is our power, our strength, and our greatest gift.

MOON CYCLE

How would your life have been different if there had been a place for you to be, a place of women, a place where, one day in your monthly stay, you were asked if it were almost time? And, if other women, somewhat older, already initiated, had begun to help you prepare?

And for many months, the women helped you during your times in the lodge to go inside yourself and consider all the experiences of your life and to reflect on them . . . if the women had helped you dream your thoughts and feelings together and to weigh them . . . so that you could come to a clearer knowing of what your life was about. And if the women had listened as

*you told them of your whole life and the sense and meaning it
held for you . . . the happenings of your whole life.*

*And, at the end of that process, after bathing and fasting and
praying, the oldest women in the lodge had come and sat in a
circle, and say that they had left an empty place . . . a place
for you. And you softly and timidly made your way to the
empty place and quietly claimed your wisdom, the wisdom of
your soul . . . How might your life be different?*

—Judith Duerk, in Circle of Stones

The first major change that a woman experiences in her
body occurs during adolescence, when she goes through
her first menstrual bleeding, or menarche. This first
initiation into womanhood has many, many different rituals
and rites of passage associated with it from cultures far
and wide. As a girl becomes a woman, often a deep sense
of self begins to emerge, and it is said that the truth of
her adult essence is born. She is known to be fertile,
abundant, and ripe.

Our culture often negates the depth of the moon cycle,
and brushes it under the carpet so to speak. For us to
truly stand in our divine feminine, we need to really heal
and transform some of the modern cultural burdens that
menstruation carries with it. In our modern-day society we
even have birth control drugs that cause a woman's body
to experience amenorrhea, skipping the menstrual period
all together. The existence of these drugs is just a small
insight into the value that we, as a culture, place on this
divine cycle with which we are gifted as part of our natural
feminine heritage. We feel it is okay to simply cancel it out
altogether for convenience. How can our true feminine

be embraced if this is the message we receive from our primary health-care providers, and from the messages we receive from our media, culture, and often even from our teachers, our mothers, and our sisters?

The menstrual cycle is known in many traditions as the body's natural monthly cleanse. During this time, we also connect to the cycles of nature—primarily those of the moon—and other women in the community, and we are able to deeply feel and intuit messages from within. This time is like a magical porthole into something untouched by men, and sacred to women and women alone. To be initiated into this process as a young woman, by the wise women, is/was an honor, and those of us who did not receive that initiation as part of our cultural heritage often experience a deep yearning for connection to the primal feminine source and power. A woman squatting on Mother Earth during the flow of her menses, regenerating the earth with her own blood, was revered as a sacred gift and connection only a woman could have. A woman initiated in her menses was taught to claim her identification with the feminine, to come to her own unique strength, wisdom, and feminine archetypal consciousness. This healing on both the individual and collective levels is an opportunity for every woman to weave her truth back into her path, her way, her journey of the goddess, the feminine, and all the future passages she will cross . . .

Ayurvedic medicine, for example, views menstruation as a cleansing time for a woman's body each month when she sheds the "ama," or toxins It is considered a time for self-healing and self-care. The quality and quantity of ama built up in the body are known to greatly affect the cycle and the experience the woman has each round of the moon. Women are said to be best in tune with the cycles of the moon if they bleed on the new moon in the winter's dark nights, and the full moon in the summer's longer days. By ridding the body of excess toxins, the menstrual time purifies the woman's body so it is not overloaded with its task and can work more easily, in the way nature intended. I personally notice more ease during menstruation if I am eating well, sleeping well, and especially expressing myself, and my emotions, freely throughout the prior month. If I am off balance, stressed, and not taking care of my needs either physically or emotionally, I will have a heightened experience of PMS, and a more challenging cycle altogether. I have learned to watch this process with more vigilance and deeper investigation. This inquiry has helped me to realize that nothing in my life goes unrecognized. Basically I cannot get away with anything anymore! I have made a commitment or contract with myself to honor my independence and to listen to my intuition. If I listen to the voice within, stay in truth, and take really good care of myself, all is flowing well within and expressed through the signs, including symptoms or lack thereof that I receive from my body.

We are so often robbed of an opportunity in our modern day to notice the waves, hormones, and various gifts our cycles can offer. We are stripped of this divine connection and cycle of nature every month, either because we simply have "turned it off" or, for some of us, because we are too depleted, due to common modern-day stressors, to even have a period (amenorrhea), or more commonly, we are simply burdened, disconnected, and annoyed by the imposition our cycle brings each month.

We are told we are grumpy, edgy, and hard to be around during our periods. Periods are often seen as messy impositions that prevent us from being sexual, fun, and outgoing. Each of us has our own beliefs and psychic pains associated with our menses, and to truly heal our sacred feminine we must acknowledge the ways in which we came to birth, and continue to carry, these negative attitudes about one of the most powerful experiences of womanhood.

I see how my entire being can go through a complete and total transformation every month. In this transformation there is a journey to something greater, which to me, is like a wise teacher. If I truly honor this inherent rhythm, I feel nourished in ways I could never have imagined. At certain times of the month I feel so expansive, talkative, outgoing, and sexual, whilst other times of the month I am quiet, contemplative, creative, introspective, and shy. These rhythms, if we honor them, have the ability to keep us real, safe, and connected to our inner fire of womanhood. They keep the female mystery and intuition alive, and they continually reveal new levels of our own divinity and inner guidance systems. The ways in which we are able to respect our cycles and energy throughout the month also teaches those around us, especially our partners, daughters, and even our sons to find a deep respect for the feminine as well.

For many of us, our first menses is terrifying, and we wish we could avoid it altogether. I was a competitive athlete and experienced a great deal of resistance and trauma with my first menses. I remember telling my mom that it had arrived, and then when she asked how she could help, I ran to my room and slammed the door, crying and hiding and wishing it would all go away. I did not know how to be in my gymnastics leotard anymore in my competitions while on my monthly cycle, and I surely would have done anything at that point to stop it from ever coming back. It took me until my mid-twenties, when I started to honor my cycle, feeling those benefits of my intuition and heightened dreams, and a connection to the moon and earth, before I ever could consider a woman's cycle a gift of the divine feminine. I was lucky to land in Boulder, Colorado, where many women do join together to honor the feminine cycles, and hold the menses in a spiritually high regard. I read books like *The Red Tent* and *Circle of Stones,* and they spoke to my heart. I learned how to practice yoga while I was menstruating in a way that nourished my body so gently and restoratively. I began teaching this to other women. I began to allow myself to rest more, write more, and give myself the gift of letting my energy and mood dictate the type of day I would have rather than following an external agenda so tightly.

There are many ways to honor ourselves throughout the month. The key is to find your way, your rituals, and the truth of your own feminine rhythm.

Visit: www.HealthWise-Woman.com/feminine for a menstrual moon practice that is delicious to experience during your moon time. Enjoy and indulge. ♀

> # HOME PRACTICE:
>
> 1.   *Write a journal entry regarding your menstrual history and the beliefs and messages you received regarding menstruation as a child.*
>
> 2.   *Create a monthly ritual that works for you. (a restorative yoga practice, a night of pampering, a women's group, a bath or spa night, a meditation.) My website can help.*
>
> www.HealthWise-Woman.com/feminine ♀
>
> 3.   *View our restorative yoga practice for menstruation online:* www.HealthWise-Woman.com/feminine ♀
>
> *Reclaiming your feminine starts here, no matter how old you are, where you have been, or where you are going . . .*

MOTHERHOOD

"Giving is the new getting."

Motherhood is the next feminine rite of passage that we will look at. It is a pinnacle porthole into one way we can find connection to our femininity and a life of service and humility. Whether we birth our own babies, adopt children in need, or mother the people in our lives—our nieces, nephews, sisters, friends, and aging parents—most of us learn the art of mothering in some way. Becoming a mother is an experience that is almost too big to put to words. We give endlessly and unconditionally even when we feel like there is nothing left to give. We grow and evolve and learn the art of selfless service, patience, and compassion like never before. We love, accept, protect, and grow in ways that nothing else can inspire. Motherhood is a true journey of the feminine flowing through us, finding the well of endless energy and unconditional love that is always there, often replenished by the simplest things like a kiss from our toddler, a brilliant school performance by our fourth grader, or even just a warm moment of openness and authenticity from our teenager.

Motherhood is signified by many different archetypes in our modern day. The queen, the empress, the goddesses of Durga, Kali, and Demeter represent many of the qualities we cultivate as mothers. Each of these archetypes speaks to each of us differently. They offer us guidance when we need it, they lend us support, camaraderie, and a sense that there have been many before us and many more to come, and that the legacy of mothers is a pool of history and future that will always be teaching us to listen, evolve, take care of ourselves, and remember.

The empress embodies the divine feminine in all her forms. She is radiant, nourishing, nurturing, accepting, and unconditional. She embodies a deep intuitive wisdom that always knows. While nourishing her own, she has an overflowing well and can nourish all living beings. The gates are always open to her heart. Her power and beauty attract others and while creating joy, she can hold the space for the children to find their inner joy. With principles of deep reverence, respect for all living beings, plants, and mother earth, living with environmental awareness, and contributing to the healing of the planet with proactive actions taken as a family. Living simply close to the earth with nature, gardens, whole foods, deep connection and communication, honoring of each individual and his/her unique gifts.

—Gerd Zeigler, in *Tarot: Mirror of the Soul: Handbook for the Aleister Crowley Tarot*

Throughout time, mothering has come with many different challenges. Mothering while husbands were at war, mothering through the Great Depression, mothering through our most recent period of the divorce epidemic, single parenting, and financial struggles, mothering children with special needs or health issues. Mothering and fathering at the same time—running the house, paying the bills while still baking the fresh pie for dinner—this is the modern-day paradigm that is pushing us to "do it all" to a greater degree than ever before. We have held the space for the children through so many phases of our history. We are so strong and capable and yet, with the changing times, mothering in the modern world has taken on a whole new meaning. Being the empowered, successful woman, and being a good mother who is available for her children, while still taking care of herself, is a new way of existence. We are the first generation to live this new paradigm and we are paving the way, stumbling occasionally, but eventually finding paths that are fulfilling, balanced, that work for us individually.

One of our biggest challenges as mothers is finding ways to take care of ourselves so our wells do not run dry, so that we have the compassion and energy to be present with our children whilst feeling inspired and fulfilled in our own lives. This is imperative, and it has taken me so long to learn—in fact I am still learning it! As a young mother I would constantly strive to be superwoman, supermom, and forgot what it took to sustain me. I would end up totally depleted and burnt out. Through the years, through evolving my inner practice and learning more about myself, I am now finally able to prioritize my own self-care, most of the time. A miracle it truly is when we can learn how to replenish the well of energy it takes to mother. This is the journey through which we not only serve our families and children but we also learn the self-respect it takes to mother while thriving in our femininity. This is the work for modern-day mothers to master: finding the balance of giving to others, while also giving back to ourselves. Listening and supporting others, while also listening inward. When we find this balance we feel successful, inspired, and engaged in part of our purpose on this earth: raising healthy individuals who will continue to work to protect the values of love and humanity, starting with themselves.

Mothering Myself

In a society preoccupied with how best to raise a child,
I'm finding a need to mesh what's best for my children
with what's necessary for a well-balanced mother.
I'm recognizing that ceaseless giving
translates into giving yourself away.
And, when you give yourself away, you're not a
healthy mother and you're not a healthy self.

So, now I'm learning to be a woman
first and a mother second.
I'm learning to just experience my own emotions
without robbing my children of their individual
dignity by feeling their emotions too.
I'm learning that a healthy child will have his own set
of emotions and characteristics that are his alone.
And, very different from mine.
I'm learning the importance of honest exchanges of
feelings because pretenses don't fool children.
They know their mother better than she knows herself.
I'm learning that no one overcomes her
past unless she confronts it.
Otherwise, her children will absorb exactly
what she's attempting to overcome.
I'm learning that words of wisdom fall on deaf
ears if my actions contradict my deeds.
Children tend to be better impersonators than listeners.
I'm learning that life is meant to be filled with as
much sadness and pain as happiness and pleasure.
And allowing ourselves to feel everything life
has to offer is an indicator of fulfillment.
I'm learning that fulfillment can't be
attained through giving myself away
But, through giving to myself and sharing with others,
I'm learning that the best way to teach my children
to live a fulfilling life is not by sacrificing my life.
It's through living a fulfilling life myself.
I'm trying to teach my children that I have a lot to learn
Because I'm learning that letting go of them
Is the best way of holding on.

—Nancy McBrine Sheehan

HOME PRACTICE

1.   *What nurtures you and refills your well? How often do you do that activity?*

2.   *Do you feel balanced as a mother? Or tired and depleted, like you have lost your sense of yourself? If the answer is tired and depleted, how can you make a shift by giving back to yourself?*

3.   *Create a NOURISH day just for you. Hire a babysitter, ask your husband or the father of your children, their grandparents, or a neighbor you trust to watch your kids, and take a retreat day just for you. You design it, you choose how to flow through the day, and please, please allow yourself to be selfish!*

MENOPAUSE

Her body was seen as magical, intuitive, and replete with a wisdom and power that was passed on from generation to generation, from grandmother to mother to daughter. Menopause was known as a time when the energy that the body had put forth during childbearing and mothering was now turned inward, and a new birth of wisdom was able to emerge from a magical place that had lain dormant. Imagine what it must have been like to live in a time when this would be your experience of aging and menopause.

Typically, anywhere between age thirty-five to fifty, a natural slowing down of hormonal output from the ovaries begins. This includes a decrease in the production of both estrogen and progesterone. The progressive changeover in the body actually takes several years, including a peri-menopausal and a post-menopausal stage.

As Dr. Christiane Northrup shares in her well-known book, *The Wisdom of Menopause*, "climacteric" is the term used to describe the biochemical process lasting six to thirteen years where periods stop and return, also commonly increasing or decreasing in duration and flow. The climacteric process is experienced on all levels: physical, emotional, and spiritual. For a woman to come through the process of menopause in a strong and healthy way, she must acknowledge what is happening on each level and work to support these changes. Caroline Myss, author of *Anatomy of the Spirit,* believes that as the menopausal years approach, the kundalini energy (energy of desire and residual power that lies coiled at the base of the spine) begins to rise. As this energy activates the chakras through which it passes, it helps release any unfinished business residing there, and this may be expressed consciously, or subconsciously, even in the form of hot flashes.

During the early stages of menopause (if it occurs naturally as opposed to hormonally induced), egg follicles begin to atrophy, which results in decreasing estrogen levels and fewer ovulations. The brain produces FSH in response to these dropping levels of estrogen. This stimulates the ovaries into overdrive. The result is increased levels of estrogen until the ovaries are finally exhausted. When this occurs, the ovaries permanently stop producing estrogen and the menses cease.

At this time there is a decrease in ovarian production of hormones and a two-fold increase in androgenic hormones from other sources. Since these androgens can act as weak estrogens, and can be precursors for estrogen production, healthy menopausal women are able to gracefully make the transition on a biochemical level.

Many aspects of life affect our experience of the world. Menopause is said to be a time when there is great potential for the wisdom and intuition of womanhood to open and blossom. Women can learn to support themselves throughout this incredibly rich period of their lives and, collectively, we will see the potential of womankind jump to new levels. The body, mind and spirit work together to create a healthy individual. From a holistic perspective, each woman can empower herself in her own healing process by looking at where imbalances lie in her lifestyle and work to bring these areas into better balance. Alignment between a woman's inner and outer worlds creates the space for health and happiness.

In Native American rituals, those women who have passed menopause or had hysterectomies—who no longer menstruate—are known to be free of the burdens and worries of possible conception and free of the role of taking care of children. Their nurturing, if given, is seen as no longer a biological imperative but, rather, a choice. These Native American wise women are said to feel validated and revered in the community and have their own lives to live, and are not bothered by the more mainstream patriarchal hype about "worthless old women." In the days of the Delphic oracle, only a postmenopausal woman could become a Pythia, a seer at the shrine. It was believed that the power of the Python

Goddess was too intense for younger women to withstand. In some Native American cultures, postmenopausal women were eligible to become tribal elders. It was these women who chose the chiefs.

As previously discussed, each individual woman must take her health into her own hands. Menopause can be a time when nature's gifts will flourish, bringing today's women greater health, happiness, and even sensuality. It is a time of rebirth—a time for transforming worn-out old patterns to make room for new ones. It is a tender time when many women redefine who they are in the world. It is truly magical to feel our personal power, to honor our needs on all levels, and to make the choices that fully support our own unique processes. As we create a new paradigm for the wise woman, the planet can and will experience a collective healing. This time of embracing our true feminine is very challenging for some, but as we step into our truth, we will receive many, many jewels in our spiritual experience. The time of menopause is a dance of liberation that holds the space for all women to emerge into embracing femininity in a deeply intimate way. In celebrating the feminine, all masks become useless and we are at one with our true nature.

Embracing the truth of our femininity has a significant outcome. This more empowered approach to honoring the cycles of the feminine has us looking forward to the pleasures of menopause—the wisdom, the intuition, and the inner knowing that come during this time of stepping fully into our wise womanhood. We can really gel with who we are, and with who we want to be in the world, for our families and for ourselves.

SEXUALITY SPEAKS

I recently held a women's group around sexuality. It is such an interesting topic to bring to a diverse group of women. We all come with our stories, traumas, challenges, and sexual bliss. We concluded, as a group, that sexuality in all its colorfulness is just plain complicated, multilayered, and a full expression of every part of ourselves. It can be so full of love, pleasure, and intimacy and yet, it can also be a place where we are shut down, where we avoid, and even a place where our insecurities are so heightened that it feels like the opposite of pleasure. Sexuality means so many things to so many women, but to clarify, here we are talking about a wide range of aspects of our sexuality: passion, orgasm, self-pleasure or masturbation, intimacy with oneself or another, penetration, oral stimulation, touch, sensuality, orientation, and exploration. Sexuality is an important part of our femininity, power, and relationships not only with others but, hopefully, also with ourselves. Throughout all of the passages we've covered referred to in this chapter, sexuality carries many stigmas and obstacles but also many rewards and much fulfillment. Our culture, for example, has defined menopause as a time when we lose our desire for sexuality and sensuality, a time when we "dry up," so to speak, when in fact, menopause can be a time when the depth of our growth, and our understanding of who we are, actually accentuate our sexual pleasure and can even bring us to the best sexual years of our lives. Our sexuality is a full expression of who we are, where we have been, and our cumulative experience as a woman. It is not constant, just as our emotions are not constant. As our cycle changes over time, so does our sexuality. Sometimes we are playful, exploratory, and experimental, and yet other times we find ourselves quiet, tired, and even shy or withdrawn.

I recently had this conversation with my partner, which may have been the most liberating conversation about sexuality I have ever had. I asked, "What if we take all pressure off each other, all expectations off of our experience, and even the pressure to please each other, to perform, to look a certain way, totally out of the picture? We can let go of performing or judging ourselves, or the other. We can say no even if we are 'supposed' to say yes, we can stop if we feel it is necessary." And bless him, he thought it was brilliant. I, for the first time, felt totally free around our sexuality together, and within myself. I felt more inspired than ever, more like my authentic self than ever, and we had an amazing shift in the intimacy of our sex life together.

I don't suggest this for everyone. Some people really need a different approach, whatever works for them and feels good to both partners. It took me almost forty years to even articulate this level of clarity and authenticity about sexuality to another human being. Sexuality is so individual, and we each have the divine right to claim our sexuality however we feel called to, but the overall point is, this is your body, your experience, and it has to feel good to you. With all of that said, sexuality can be a beautiful path to ecstasy with yourself or another. Our bodies are designed to express high amounts of pleasure (read on for more in Secret #8, "The Pleasure Principle") and it is each individual's journey to find out how that works best for her.

What were the messages you received as a child around sex? How about around masturbation? Do you feel empowered around your sexuality, or is it challenging, terrifying, even traumatic—or do you experience both ends of this spectrum?

MEET DEB

Deb Rubin is an individual and couples therapist specializing in relationships and sexuality in Boulder Colorado. Her work as a sexuality specialist is based on helping men and women to access the deepest potential of their human existence. Deb believes sexuality is a deep, interconnected part of who we are. Sexuality can be a hard subject for people to talk about, and she is able to give people the invitation to open up in a safe place. Increasing the depth of their relationship with themselves is another place women can become their own witnesses. Deb shares: "Each version of ourselves, and our sexuality, needs a voice to be fully integrated. When women have the opportunity to explore their sexual history, and the early messages they have been given, they can see how these beliefs impact their sexual expression to date." Women sharing their sexual stories with other women in groups, has proven to be a valuable piece of Deb's work. She says, "Often sexuality can feel isolating, intimidating, and vulnerable. Sharing opens the connection between women, and therefore within the self."

Deb recommends many ways to make sexuality part of a regular practice for ourselves, leading us down a path of greater self-intimacy and connection. Here are some of her recommended practices:

- *Meditation:* practice meditation or some type of contemplative practice to connect with the inner self.
- *Ritual:* dates with yourself are a helpful way to create the time and space to tend to the body connection.
- *Sensuality (however that is interpreted by the individual):* consciously waking up the senses, as in self-massage, enhancing smells, tastes, and sounds that feel good.
- *Self-inquiry:* spending time witnessing, journaling, and learning more about oneself and one's sexual expression.
- *Self-love:* enjoying self-love, or even just the intention of self-love.
- *Safety:* creating safety and trust, giving yourself permission to learn to express, discovering what is true for you.

You can find an inspiring interview with Deb Rubin on the Health Wise website: www.HealthWise-Woman.com/feminine ♀

FEMININE EMPOWERMENT

As we return to these natural rhythms of the feminine inherent in a woman's life cycles and sexual expression, we are gifted with so much insight and grace. We can begin to ride the waves with intention, instead of resistance. We can see that these rites of passage are there to give us permission to find our truth and our power—to share ourselves in a way that serves the greater collective healing and transformation of how we see the feminine today. This work is critical, and we are at a critical time. As with any tradition, there are always gems or gifts with which we move forward, as well as some old ways that we have outgrown and need to release.

Embracing the feminine is not about living a life that is outdated or pretending to be something or somewhere we are not, but rather it's an opening into the ways in which we can truly thrive in the modern day, while embracing all the parts of ourselves, and keeping alive the legacy left for womanhood that will continue to serve our planet. Embracing the feminine is about remembering on a cellular level how to move and dance in the world in a way that fully honors ourselves. This is the truth. Our world, our planet, and our people need healing—feminine healing—and gentleness in order to remember the divine balance—the strongest healing on the planet.

EXTERNAL
AWAKENING

SECRET # 5

A Path Of Practice

Love is the great miracle cure. Loving ourselves works miracles in our lives.

—Louise Hay

This chapter is dedicated with gratitude to Bri Maya Twari, for her loving devotion and contribution to the field of health, healing, and spiritual awakening.

The word "sadhana," refers to the daily ways in which we illuminate who we are with each act we engage in. As we hone in on our daily rituals, practices, and ways to connect more deeply with the oneness space inside, we find that life begins to be infused with a mindfulness and awareness that accentuates our experiences throughout the day-to-day.

"Sadhana" is a sanskrit word with the root "sadh," a verb root which means to reclaim the power within our own hearts. This can be the power to serve, the power to connect, the power to heal, or the power to uplift. Sadhana is not limited to the time we spend on our yoga mats, or in meditation, but rather as we practice our sadhana, it begins to permeate our day-to-day activities, work, chores, relationships, and obligations.

We use the word "practice" because this skill of sadhana starts with our practices, our daily rituals, and our connection to our innermost hearts. We do need to "practice" this. We do need to "practice" listening to our intuition, being mindful, and truly living in the moment. Much of our culture is disconnected from this type of living. Unfortunately, for many of us, it is not coming naturally anymore. It may even start out feeling like completely foreign territory as we begin.

As we see yoga communities explode in popularity around the country, and the same with the number of people who study with spiritual teachers, practice meditation, and go on retreats, we can see our immense need and desire to reconnect with a centered way of being that we have lost track of in our modern world. We are craving this as a culture, yet many of us are not sure how to find our way back to the internal joy of living that is beyond the material, deeper than our societal status or whatever external recognition we may or may not receive. What I speak of here is our divinity, our spiritual connection, and our relationship with ourselves. We can then start the journey of beginning to remember the divine love that is available to us in every breath, every moment of gratitude, and every gaze with which we connect to one another.

Whether or not you are someone who believes in a higher spirit, God, or cosmic universal forces, and even if you would rather consider yourself agnostic or atheist, you can still practice love, or being a better, more aware, and more integrated person. Listening to your thoughts and deepening your relationship with yourself is a gift no matter what your spiritual orientation is. Finding a daily practice or practices that align(s) with these beliefs in you is important and it is one of the most consistently healing tools you can give yourself.

DAILY PRACTICES

The question is, what does it take to create sadhana, or practice, in our own lives, and how do we sustain a daily practice for ourselves while maybe even inspiring other people along the way? The good news is that there are many, many ways to practice. There are infinite ways to connect with yourself, and many ways to create daily rituals to fulfill yourself in your daily life. It is really about finding the ways that inspire you, move you, and are sustainable for you. Personally, my favorites are yoga, chanting, journaling, reading the Tarot, and doing visioning practices similar to the ones you have been doing throughout the previous chapters. There is not one way or one structure to use that is better than another. It's more important to find practices that you look forward to.

FIND JOY AND FULFILLMENT IN YOUR PRACTICE

It is important that your daily practice speaks to you, inspires you, and leaves you feeling satisfied, fulfilled, and content. If this is not the case, then you will most likely encounter resistance within yourself to doing it regularly. Resistance around making the time to practice is a challenge for some, but the challenge is made so much easier if you enjoy your practice.

I love yoga. Yoga asana (postures linked with breath) feels so good in my body that if I go for more than a few days without them, I feel myself screaming out for yoga. The philosophy and the teachings that include the yamas and niyamas, and the beautiful Tantric philosophy, are also ways that I strive to live. I resonate with the yogic path and principles. When I chant in Sanskrit, I feel a deep sense of freedom on the inside. Large amounts of energy/prana move through me and it is super nourishing. My radiance and vitality are absolutely connected to my yoga practice. I enjoy vigorous practice at some times of the month, and other times I really enjoy a more fluid yin or restorative practice (similar to the moon practice listed in Secret # 4 for the menstrual cycle). I customize my yoga practice for how my energy is, how much time I have, and what I feel in my body. I like to practice with others in class, and I also like to practice in my house, to my own music, in my own sacred space. Yoga clears my mind, and reminds me of my essence, truth, and purpose. It is an integral part of my work as a coach, as a nutritionist, and as a mother. It helps me with patience and finding my center. I am reminded to breathe, to take the higher road, and to take care of myself.

I also do well with a sitting practice to still my mind and connect to the deeper waves of my internal dialogue. I enjoy using this time to resolve inner conflict by listening to my intuition, breathing, and feeling my body temple express its wisdom. Sometimes that quiet space to sit in silence and stillness grounds me like nothing else I have ever known. I get to witness my mind chatter and separate the mind chatter from the voices of my higher self. I finish feeling more myself, and more centered and grounded. I often have openings to creative moments and a truer sense of self-love and self-compassion. And I frequently notice an overall sense of relaxation and calmness come over me.

CREATE A SUSTAINABLE PRACTICE

Sustainability is what will create the long-term results that we are all looking for in our lives. I have learned that if I get a little too rigid, or over committed, I usually lose the ability to keep my practice flowing. Creating the type of daily practice that you can follow through on even in a busy day is important. That, for me, may involve a five to ten minute meditation, or a quiet cup of tea in my meditation space while I read my Tarot.

If I really commit to a longer practice for a period of time, which at times I do, then I need to make sure to schedule it into my day before the time sneaks away. Practice is something that is more effective with more consistency, more regularity, and more, well, practice! When my obstacles or resistance come up, I turn to friends, teachers, or community for support to keep on moving forward. Sometimes we just need to re-evaluate what it is we want our practice to bring to our lives. The value of daily practice over time is priceless and will shift your life experience. This may be enough to keep you inspired and on track. I find it helpful to write down the qualities my life is infused with when I practice regularly, and then keep this list somewhere available to me to read over when I come up against my blocks.

FOLLOW YOUR RHYTHM

One of the ways I play with my practice that I find enjoyable is to notice how it fluctuates with my own rhythms. My monthly cycle and the seasonal cycles of the year are big influences on me combined with the general inspiration they offer me within my practice. I notice that during the cold, dark winter I enjoy meditating by candlelight, journaling, and being more in the quiet, dark space—going inward. Then in the light of the summer, I am more expansive and may practice yoga outside on my porch in the early morning sun, or even sit by the creek and meditate. I move more, and sit less, in the expansiveness of summer, and hibernate more in the darkness of winter.

Our menstrual cycles are times of similar flow within each month. We expand during pre-ovulation and ovulation, and we contract during post-ovulation and menstruation. Knowing this, can help you to design your daily practice, and to better understand the flow of your own organic rhythm, which is a very important awareness to develop as a woman to increase your health.

Creating a variety of practices to match your energy, or finding classes that match your energy during your own fluctuations, is soothing to your femininity and flow. Daily practice can and will meet you right where you are.

CALL IN YOUR SUPPORT

As most of us progress along a path to higher consciousness and awareness in our daily lives, we find ourselves, seeking and creating community with like-minded people who have values and ideals that are similar to our own. Through these relationships we are able to keep each other uplifted, discuss our personal successes and obstacles, and share in the joy of living mindful lives together. This has been a common thread between communities all across time and across the planet. People often come together because they have similar beliefs and values.

I personally cherish my yoga community, and the women in my life who I can turn to, to create ritual, to participate in collective spiritual practice, and to discuss where I am at and what I am experiencing. It has become such an integral part of our social time together and of our celebrations, and one of the key ways in which we can share the beauty of the feminine. One of the very cool offerings I've created for you is a virtual community through the Health Wise website (www.HealthWise-Woman.com), where you can connect with women all around the country who are working on some of the same practices you are, and are interested in becoming more active in their health and their view of themselves, and connecting with women just like you, creating a wonderful support system nationwide! ♀

CREATING SACRED SPACE

Whether you have an extraordinary space in your house, or a tiny magical corner that calls to you, it is important and helpful to create a sacred space where you can do your daily practice. This may involve an altar space, a journaling space, a meditation cushion, a yoga mat, a favorite window chair, or a place where you have objects and affirmations that remind you of parts of yourself you want to bring forth or qualities you wish to emulate; or it may even have a vision board, vision box, or affirmations board. Candles can help create the ambiance that helps you drop in, as can music, either that you listen to or play yourself, to soothe you as you practice (depending on the style of practice you prefer), and whatever else makes it a comfortable, beautiful, and workable space for you to use.

I find that I settle into one arrangement for a while, and then later I totally redo my space when I feel inspired. Sometimes it is really simple and empty, and other times it is more full. I ride out my calling to create the space I yearn for in the moment, whatever that is. As women, we know how things can change for us. Sometimes we want it one way and then "poof!"— what we want changes. Trust this in yourself, as there is no right or wrong way to create your space. It could be anything from a nook under the stairs, to a tree house, to an entire yoga room that is made just for you. The most important thing is that it is yours, and that it calls to you.

SHARING YOUR PRACTICE

As we find our connection and strengthen our relationship with ourselves, others do notice. "How do you do it? What are you up to in your life that is working so well for you? How are you looking and feeling so radiant, vibrant, and inspired in your life?" These are the questions people begin to ask us, because the truth is, it is obvious. When we live this way, we begin to shine, and it is contagious. How inspiring is that? The more we can take care of ourselves, be selfish in a healthy way with our own practice, and enjoy the time to connect inward, the more we can give back, both by doing and by just being. We are better partners, mothers, teachers, and friends when our well of self-love and sadhana is full, and consistently so. We can listen more effectively to others, we can share more articulately, and we can love more fully because we are in touch with our own self-love on a deeper level.

Just today I was in the grocery store line and a friend approached me. He said, "You look radiant, whatever it is you are doing these days, keep doing it. You are glowing!" For me, this is sharing my practice with others. Maybe I share the details and maybe I just smile and say thank you, and that is enough to shift someone who is having a tough day or needing to be uplifted. Maybe my practice shows up at dinner when I defuse an argument between my two boys (brothers!), or maybe it is that I am a more effective coach. Either way, it is worth the effort, and it does not go unnoticed. Diligence and consistency are on our side.

Creating your daily practices, and living them on a daily basis, is an enormous gift that you are giving your soul. It may seem like you are going through the motions at first, it may feel uncomfortable and even a bit silly, but the benefits will soon show up. Stay with it and trust the process. There are many, many books, documentaries, and resources for you to find inspirational teachers, methods, and communities to join with. Some of these have a spiritual orientation of a certain type and some of them do not. Align yourself with what resonates with you. Your way is the ultimate practice for YOU. This will help you to keep yourself centered, even, and balanced, even when life throws you twists and turns that feel like too much, too scary, too challenging. There is a list of some practices to consider at the end of this chapter, and on the interactive website at www.HealthWise-Woman.com/pathofpractice. I hope you enjoy some of my favorites. ♀

MEET HOLLY

Holly is a 30-year-old woman who lives in Denver, Colorado. Holly is a dedicated school teacher who works a lot! Her day-to-day life can be hectic with the demands of her career, and she often gets overwhelmed and burnt out. Holly enjoys activities like yoga, running, being outdoors, and spending time with friends and family. Holly came to me for support around her relationship with food and her eating disorder, and for help with how to better manage her health within her busy schedule. After we worked together and got the "nuts and bolts" of healthy eating worked out, Holly was still struggling internally with self-control, stress, and being caught up in an overachieving lifestyle, leaving her feeling depleted. I taught her to meditate and she began to implement a daily practice into her routine. Let me add, meditation was brand new to her at the time.

Holly shares: "Practicing daily helps me stay connected to myself. I am more grounded, more mindful. When I do Yoga three days in a row, I am much more positive. I am better at relating to others, more present in general. I stay connected to who I am."

Holly would like to take it deeper, learning new strategies, breathing techniques, and little things throughout the day. She says, "I am considering maybe doing a yoga training, teaching others, and deepening into the practice in many facets. Sharing with others, teaching others, friends and family… watching the domino effect in my life and with others is really satisfying."

Holly feels the difference in life and recognizes the changes:. "After hitting coming up from rock bottom with bulimia, then I realized that who I am, and what I am doing, has meaning. I see how far I have come, and I realize there is so much more out there for me."

Working with a supportive coach, and seeing that we all progress along our journey, with the right tools to deal with what is arising, has kept Holly hopeful that she can continue to shift her old patterns into new ones that serve her today.

"I still catch myself in negative self-talk, but way less often. At first I hated my body all the time, now I am learning to accept my athletic build and appreciate it for all it gives me. Daily practice helps me to catch the negative self-talk. Let go and accept more now."

Here are a few of Holly's favorite practices:

- *Yoga practice*
- *Meditation*
- *Immersing myself in mindfulness*
- *Reading Byron Katie, Eckhart Tolle, and many other inspiring authors*
- *Sessions with Sue*

- *Talking and sharing with others in the community of like mind*

By the time this book gets into your hands, Holly will have completed her yoga-teacher training, and she will be preparing to teach others yoga, one of her passions. She is already inspired by her new community, her fellow yoga teacher trainees, and is now taking even more time to practice, leaving work earlier in the evening to allocate the time she needs to take care of herself, nourish herself, and breathe. This has been a huge transformation for Holly.

HOME PRACTICES

1. *Cultivate a daily practice that inspires you and practice it daily for 1 week. Make the commitment to yourself and see what happens. Schedule this into your day, literally into your calendar! I recommend either first thing in the AM, or right before bed.*

2. *Create a sacred space in your life where you can go to be in your daily practice. This is an expression of you, to remind you of your intentions and your heart-centered living.*

3. *Share your practice with another person. Maybe they will join you in committing to their practice for 7 days with you, or maybe you can just share with them how it is going along the way. The buddy system makes everything easier.*

4. *Download a daily practice of your choice from the plentiful offerings on my website.* www.HealthWise-Woman.com/pathofpractice. *Here you can browse the offerings and find something that works for you.* ♀

SECRET # 6

Heart and Soul Communication

Love is our true destiny. We do not find the meaning of life by ourselves alone - we find it with another.

—Thomas Merton

As we open, trust, and expand into ourselves more and more fully throughout our own personal journeys, it is natural to want to express ourselves in our communications in such a way that our truth and hearts can emerge to share with another person. It is a true soul yearning to share ourselves in our relationships, and even to maybe be fully understood by others. Just as we long to watch a beautiful sunset with another person, share laughter, or the moment when our child takes her first step, sharing the intimacy of our inner experience with one another can bring a sense of connection, joy, and freedom to our relationships.

Our authentic selves grow and become so much more accessible and noticeable to each of us through all of our personal work, but how can we intimately share our authentic selves with others? Our partners, friends, and families are an integral part of the health and support in our daily lives, and yet often one of the most difficult challenges many of us have is to really be able to open ourselves into our relationships without all of our old paradigms and automatic ways of communicating running the show. Often we are so caught up in our own stories and thoughts that we miss these amazing opportunities to reach outside of ourselves, connect with another person, and find the beauty in the right here and right now—together.

What would it be like if our communication in our relationships were another vehicle into our personal growth, and another opportunity to stay in the present moment? If our communication is similar to our meditation, one that we share with one another, think of the colorful moments we can embrace with each other. Imagine the possibility of allowing the art of heart and soul communication to be an integral part of our own growth as well as the growth of our relationships and communities . . .

SPEAKING THE TRUTH

Let's face it, as women most of us have not been brought up to speak our truth. Even if good intentions were put forth for many of us as young children, the ability to be authentic, to speak our truth, and even to state our needs is not something most women are able to do naturally. Most of us have needed a lot of attentiveness around communication skills, and, in many cases, even coaching, counseling, or spiritual practice to learn to speak our truth in the moment. Our culture is inherently repressive when it comes to authentic communication, as are many other modern-day cultures. Women have been taught for generations worldwide to avoid "rocking the boat," and instead to "people please," putting ourselves and our own opinions and desires aside. One of the most exciting aspects of the new times afoot, in which the collective consciousness is beginning to evolve and heal all over the planet, is that our authentic communication is starting to strengthen. We are being called to make a shift for women everywhere, and it begins with us as individuals. It is a challenge that brings so much liberation and freedom into our relationships, but also we must overcome our conditioning and patterning that is often running, and prevent it from taking over. We may need to face large amounts of fear, and sometimes even panic, as we become willing to "own" our experiences and share what is true, even if it may not "please" others. We may have to jump off that perceived cliff and know that within our fear there is a well of trust—trust that our relationships can deepen, our friendships can become more full, and our partnerships can transcend to new levels of intimacy and connection. With that said, there is always a chance that some relationships will fall away. The relationships that do not serve us for the long term, or those that are not set up to handle the non-superficial aspects of life may not survive.

The beauty of speaking the truth in the moment is that we are able to let go of the stories, the patterns of victimhood, and empower ourselves to share the moment-to-moment experiences that make up life in its most radiant forms. We can reclaim the present moment in communication as a meditation that keeps us centered, grounded, and attuned to our inner experience. Our "inner listening" skills become even more refined, just as they do in any spiritual practice, because we have to stay with each rising sensation, emotion, and thought in order to share it with another person. This helps us to stay authentic to what is our truth in the moment, rather than finding ourselves caught up in the old tapes and stories in our minds that may even be totally outdated and irrelevant.

COMMUNICATION AS MEDITATION

Communication as a meditation is all about staying in the present moment, from moment to moment, throughout our connections and communications with one another. As you begin to open and share, your physical body, mainly your senses, is the perfect tool, and one that you always have with you as your own barometer for each experience or communication. The physical sensations and thoughts that arise in the present moment are reminders that we can use to inspire our communications.

Authentic, heart-centered communication based on experiencing the present moment.

1.   **State the present physical sensation.**

If you can start with this as a practice, it will open the door to more authentic communication. Here are some examples.

"My throat is tight and I feel tingling in my arms."

"I feel energized, tingly, and warm."

As we share the arising sensations with another person, he or she can then have a deeper insight into what our experience is, from the inside out.

I use this technique with my women's groups, and it has proven to be a beautiful way to open the doors to our hearts so we can connect deeply with each other. As we practice this style of communication, it can at first feel awkward, as many of us are used to either shutting down completely, or going right to our habitual stories (our monkey minds). Sometimes when we are beginning this practice it is even challenging just to articulate what exactly the physical sensations are that we are experiencing in the present moment. It can take a bit of practice. Here we have a new emerging pattern to work with. Communication as meditation is a very different approach for most of us. Like anything new, it can feel awkward, strange, or even uncomfortable at first. It gets easier, and we can form positive habits with more and more practice.

2.   Share the emotional sensation.

As we move from body sensation to emotion, we are already grounded in the present and then the emotion that is arising is more relevant to the present, and more authentic to the present situation. For example:

"I feel scared to share myself with you, and I feel like running away."

"I am excited, and happy to be here with you."

Moving from sensation to emotion is setting the stage for a communication that is more readily understood, with fewer projections, fewer mind games, and decreased childish behavior. Heart and soul communication is grounded in truth, the adult self, and rational processes in which the individual is taking ownership of his/her experience and sharing it in a way that can be understood. Have you ever caught yourself bringing a past experience or emotion to a conversation that has absolutely no relevance to the current conversation? Maybe you were angry with your spouse a week prior and all of a sudden that is the displaced emotion that is running the show. Meanwhile, your spouse is totally confused. We have all been there, and the truth is, the cumulative effect of this is not so healthy. If we can express our feelings, thoughts, inner experience (positive or negative) more in the moment, we are freer and more clear, and our quality of communication is much more effective. Then we can move into the mind/thought portion of experience with a solid foundation.

3.   **Share your thoughts.**

"I imagine that you are angry at me. I feel sorry, and afraid you will want to leave."

"I am thinking that I really enjoy you and your company, and I am excited to take this adventure with you."

The suffering that we each individually experience also has a collective element to it—our respective individual experiences share common threads. For some reason most of us are taught something different from this truth—we're taught that our suffering is uniquely our own and that it's something to be ashamed of. This is why it is hard to open up and share the truth of the moment.

I was working through something with my partner recently, and I was so terrified to share. As I got closer, and closer, a feeling of intense nausea took over. I felt like I literally might vomit, the fear was so intense. I finally said, "I feel like I might vomit, and I am terrified to talk about this with you. I feel vulnerable and raw."

Before we even got to the heart of the matter, he heard me, saw me, and saw how hard it was for me to open up in this area. He listened without judgment. To me, this is intimacy. Along with all the beautiful, heart-centered lovemaking and affectionate stuff, there is the hard, raw, exposing stuff that is challenging to share and hard to speak about. But during this recent conversation with my partner, as I let the interaction settle, and as I watched how intently he could listen, understand, and almost feel my experience, a new level of trust was born. I experienced a new level of pure intimacy, felt a deep release of tension within myself, and ended up feeling even closer to him than ever before.

I have also tried this with my teenager when we have a challenge communicating. We often experience blame and judgment with each other. As an alternative, I can patiently sit, listen, receive his comments, and then reply via my physical experience. This gives him a reflection of how he is being heard in the moment. For example, I might share:

"I hear your anger. When I hear your angry comments towards me, I notice my stomach contracts and I feel hot all over. I feel sad and angry. I imagine that you are frustrated with me."

Heart and soul communication may be one-sided communication or it may eventually become reciprocal, with two people "practicing" this together. Either way, this is about *your* communication, *your* authentic expression, and *you* sharing yourself because *you* desire a deeper connection. We can never control another person, but it is imperative that we create our own experience in our communications. The healing happens as we keep tuning in more and more deeply to ourselves, using our bodies, senses, and emotions as our teachers.

AUTOMATIC RESPONSES

Watching for your automatic responses in your communication will give you a lot of information about yourself. We all have them—they are habitual, ingrained parts of our own suffering. We get something out of them, which is why they have been there for so long, but making a shift is imperative to awaken our health and improve our communication skills. There are a few common automatic responses that you may connect with, or yours may be more unique. Either way, witness and observe, so that you can be the one in charge, driving the ship, choosing how to share in the moment. Being taken over by the automatic will not serve you in your higher health and consciousness.

1.   **Righteousness**

Mmmm. Feeling right is fabulous sometimes . . . but is it really? I have worked with this one for years. I have even been told I should have been a lawyer because I can always prove myself right. When I really look at this pattern in myself honestly, I have one word for it: YUCK!

Who wants to be the righteous one? Not me! But it is so ingrained in many of us. Our conflicts are often a who's right, who's wrong conversation. Surrendering righteousness is tough. It is like getting naked in front of a whole room of people who are just staring at you.

Remember the character of Fonzarelli in *Happy Days*? He could not say the words "I am wrong." He would fumble and fumble, because he was "too cool" to be wrong. Well, many of us have some of that going on, but let's agree, when we can own it, take it, and admit we are wrong, or at least not absolutely right, things really open up with the person we are talking with. Our egos can take a rest (thank God) and we can be humans, who are sometimes wrong, and we are better able to see the big picture.

2. **Excuses**

Do you ever watch yourself making an excuse for no reason at all? "Sorry I'm late, but the traffic was HORRIBLE!" Rather than the truth: "Sorry I am late, but I just wasn't on top of things and I was running behind." Are excuses just another way you separate yourself from other people? Excuses don't do us much good, and they surely are not part of practicing authentic communication. Sometimes they are just habits, or sometimes we are just plain scared to tell the truth. "I feel ashamed to say it, but I am late, and I really need to work on my time management." Ahhh, doesn't that feel so much better? It may be harder, but there you are again, being real, being true, and letting another person see you!

Life without excuses would be interesting, and maybe even comical. Why is it we are so afraid to tell the truth? Our minds often tell us someone may judge us, dislike us, or even talk badly about us. What is the trade-off? The truth is, if we own it our sincerity is felt by the other person. We are most often not judged but, instead, recognized for speaking from our hearts, and people learn to trust us and know us for being honest. Excuses are a dead-end road in the world of authentic communication, and they are also a sure way to give away our power and remain the one who lost in the situation. Excuses can be so common in our way of expression that we barely even notice ourselves making them. The *"I don't have time,"* the *"I don't have the money,"* and the *"I am too tired"* are really products of our lack of commitment, which is fine, but let's just say it how it is. When someone says to you, *"I can't make it work because it is really just not a priority for me at this time,"* there is a feeling of completion. When there is something you really want, let's face it: you make the time. Challenge yourself to an excuse-free life. Be authentic, and share what is really true. *"Sorry, but I am just not that interested in your project for reasons X, Y, and Z."* The truth really does set you free.

3. **The Blame Game**

How often are we tempted to blame the other person, point the finger, and essentially, give our power away? That is really what blaming is. This is not to say that everyone involved doesn't have his or her part, but *you* are only able to take responsibility for *yours.* If we are constantly pointing the finger, we are not reflecting on our own part, and what we are doing is playing the victim. Playing the victim really never gets us anywhere. It's a huge blow-off to being present and taking ownership. It is time to be willing to stand tall within ourselves and remember that we are in the driver's seat here. Blaming is giving away your power to another person. Own it, sister! Free yourself from the blame game.

BREAKING FREE

All in all, our communication is the primary way in which we move from the internal world to the external world. It is how we share ourselves, how we connect with our families, friends, and partners. Refining your communication to a style that is a true expression of your deepest heart self is a wonderful way to open and transform. You will have more amazing moments with the people around you, and more deep, authentic experiences of exposing who you truly are from the inside out. The richness of life will unfold before you with grace and beauty, and others will be able to join you in that unfolding. What a gift!

MEET DAYNA

Dayna is a 30-year-old woman with whom I have worked for many years. She enjoys design and is really good at it (in fact, she designed the cover of this book), and she also has passions in dance, yoga, and somatic psychotherapy.

Dayna and I took a communication workshop together (a first for both of us at the time) from a local teacher on a retreat in Costa Rica (neither of us had ever been on a retreat before, either), and we dove into the work in parallel. Dayna says that after working with authentic communication for a while she now finds she is able to drop into the present moment, slow down, and sense what is going on in the now. This enables her to avoid falling back into old communication patterns like assumptions, projections, or basing what she is saying in the past or future instead of "getting real" with what is actually going on!

Bringing this work to her relationships is a continual practice of keeping it in her consciousness and awareness, as it takes practice to communicate this way consistently.

She has learned that listening is being present enough to listen both inward, to yourself, and outward, to the other person. She works on not getting caught up in her own stories. This is like making an offering to another human being that is about listening, noticing, and really wanting to be listened to. Giving and receiving this way feels like a gift.

As Dayna has opened to her authentic self, she has been able to build a really strong foundation for all of her relationships—a foundation of the practice of allowing her own authentic experience in the moment to have space and then giving voice to it.

"I was just noticing the little things that bother me in subtle ways, that accumulate over time, can get caught and stuck. The third body, 'the relationship body,' when it gets stuck, can lead to the bigger triggers. Being able to process through the things that could eventually become obstacles is like preventative medicine to any relationship, to release stuck emotions before they accumulate and become bad relationship patterns."

Dayna believes that we are often trained from a very young age to meet certain expectations of one another, which often means not expressing our truth, blaming, and/or projecting. Essentially we need to learn the tools and techniques to re-train ourselves to feel safe with our authentic selves and experiences.

"*Since doing this work, there is a deeper body-mind connection for me that is more integrated. Sensations, emotions, and thoughts are more cross-communicated and there is a deep listening and attunement to myself and my physicality. I enjoy listening and trusting myself, dropping into the present, like a meditation quality in day-to-day life, observing, witnessing.*"

Studying Hakomi (a body-centered psychotherapy) has also helped Dayna drop into the art of allowing. Yoga and other awareness practices, such as meditation and dance, have also been big contributors to getting comfortable in her body and the present experience of being.

Dayna has made major breakthroughs in her relationships using the tools of authentic communication. She feels more and more comfortable speaking her truth and her needs, and sharing herself.

HOME PRACTICE

1.   *With a good friend, partner, or family member, practice heart-and-soul communication: physical sensation, emotion, thought, in that order, as described above.*

2.   *Write down your most frequent automatic ways of communicating, and watch for them throughout your day. Begin an awareness practice around authentic communication, working with shifting out of your automatic ways of communicating, toward more intentional ways of communicating.*

(We have a great worksheet for this on the Health Wise website. www.HealthWise-Woman.com/heartandsoul) ♀

3.   *Challenge yourself to an excuse-free day or week. Instead of making excuses, speak the truth, own your experience, and see what happens. This is a great practice that will help you to be more authentic in your connection with others.*

Free downloads available.
www.HealthWise-Woman.com/heartandsoul ♀

SECRET #7

Vibrant Wealth, Vibrant Health

If you have debt I'm willing to bet that general clutter is a problem for you too.

–Suze Orman

FINANCIAL AFFIRMATION

I now claim total fulfillment of my potential.

May I be an instrument of love.

I now call in the highest and best that I have to give the world.

Let it be made manifest in and through me.

I now claim financial mindfulness and mastery. I align the power of my subconscious mind with the principles of wealth and prosperity. I am a source of abundance and wealth. I am a creator of abundance and wealth. I am a sustainer of abundance and wealth. Prosperity flows through me from the creative well within me. I use my time, my money, my resources, and my attention wisely. I use these in the name of love and compassion. I contribute to my family, my community, and the world. I celebrate the creation of pleasurable, lavish, opulent, and extraordinary abundance.

I say YES to life!

I am now in line with the divine plan for myself and for my family.

I allow the principles of life to establish harmony, starting with me. I open to see the great opportunities emerging as I release the past, open to full empowerment,

and focus on the best in myself.

L earning to be empowered, in charge, and wise about our wealth and prosperity as women in the twenty-first century is a challenge many of us have faced. I have become clear that our financial stress and struggle have a huge long-term impact on our health, which is why I have included this topic here in *Health Wise*. This chapter is designed to inspire you to take charge of your finances, prosperity, and overall wealth so you can feel the benefits all the way down to the core of your health. Depending on the experiences and beliefs of the women who came before you, this history can create a ripple effect of various beliefs and energies such as lack mentality, confusion, and/or shame. Despite how far we have come socially as women today, in the area of money we commonly give away our power, and succumb to fear, denial, and even to our shadows. This is not our fault. It is simply due to the fact that it is relatively new for women to be working for money, managing our own prosperity, and taking charge of how we want to relate to our own abundance in the world independent of men. Women today are paving the way. With that said, we, as empowered women, can take our healing into our own hands and find ways to make a shift, heal the old paradigms that are not working, and move forward doing something new. Recent studies show that in 40%

of households, women today now earn more than their husbands. In an article published by the Wall Street Journal, it was projected that by the year 2030, women will control 2/3 of the nation's wealth if the current financial trend continues. With that said, women also tend to save less, invest less, and spend more. It is also critical to look at how this money story began and changed over time. In other words, what happened?

THE SHE HISTORY OF MONEY

As mentioned earlier, historically women were more connected to spirit, the cycles of the moon, divine intuition, and prayer. There was a time when not a seed was planted without a ritual, not a harvest went by without acknowledging the goddess at work providing a connection between heaven and earth. Money didn't even exist in its physical form the way it does now. Money was simply the physical connection between spirit and earth. Each year the great Mother Earth strived to provide everything mankind needed to survive, and we could track energy exchange through the trade of commodities. When money took its physical form, around 2500 B.C., it became the connection between the material and the spiritual planes. After the infiltration of the Christian church, and the Industrial Revolution, money lost its connection with the spiritual realm and became strictly a means of exchange, as well as a commodity used to define a person's class, educational status, and overall material wealth. Eventually, in the spiritual world, money even developed a somewhat evil reputation that is still prevalent for some of us today. To the spiritual seeker, money often represented greed, materialism, and even corruption.

Since the turn of the century, women have come a long way. We have achieved the right to vote, the right to divorce a man on the same grounds upon which a man can divorce a woman, and the opportunity to graduate from a university; we have empowered ourselves around birth control, pregnancy, and childbirth. Women have taken back our power in so many ways, but somehow money is still an area where we often live in the dark, handing our power over to men, staying uninvolved, in fear and confusion, and keeping ourselves in a general malaise around money. Why is money such a hard area for us to feel strong and empowered in? Who were our role models, and what is our lineage around money as women?

When we examine our own personal money histories, and the collective history of women and money, the answers to some of these questions are right there in front of our eyes. In the big picture, women just recently became official earners in our society. Gaining the rights to open a bank account, earn credit, and apply for a loan are all still relatively new advances. But throughout all the changes outside the home, many, many in-home roles have remained the same. It has only been over the last twenty years, during which the divorce rate has risen to nearly fifty percent, that women have made up close to half of the workforce. With this trend, and with women increasingly acting as sole providers as well as managers of household finances, we now have not only the incentive but also the drive borne of necessity to figure out the money question. Even as these monumental changes have taken place we are often left with what appear to be only two choices: either we act just as the women before us did, or "rebel" and find a different way. Neither route is going to serve us particularly well in the financial world. What we have to do is gradually unravel our own personal belief systems and paradigms around money and begin to move forward in creating new ones that empower us. This can create a huge domino effect of healing for generations to come!

I had a really enlightening conversation with my ninety-year-old British grandmother, whom I called Nan, right before she died. Nan was chatting with my sister, my cousin, and me one afternoon after a good strong cup of British tea and some biscuits. She knew she was sick, and her energy was slowly beginning to dwindle. She was definitely the queen of our family, and had always been concerned for us girls, particularly with regard to how and when we would each "settle down." Nan had concerns about us being on our own, alone in the world, and like all grandmothers, always wanted to see more great-grandchildren ASAP! "As a young woman and mother Nan had not had a driver's license (and didn't obtain one until in her mid 50's) and had spent very little time in the work force, balancing a checkbook, or participating in any of the financial decisions for the family." During this conversation, my cousin, a successful lawyer, elucidated the generation gap for us by explaining,

"Nan, the difference is that when you were young and riding on the back of [Grandpa's] scooter around town, you were looking to merge with a man who could 'take care of you.' You needed each other in a different way. We, as empowered young businesswomen who live alone, or with our children, run our households fairly smoothly and do not need a male, so to speak, to drive us to the grocery store, pay our bills, or take care of us in that way—we can actually merge with a man because we want to, solely because they accent who we are, and simply enhance how we want to live. We can be picky because there is no rush when we are fairly self-sufficient."

Our dear Nan had a blank expression in her eyes and paused for a moment. I think she realized in that moment that something had changed for womankind as a whole. Of course she went back to drinking her tea and offered us more biscuits, as per her usual, and we all kind of chuckled to ourselves. But this was a moment when my own personal money legacy lit up and flashed before my eyes . . . wow, there it was! I, along with many women, am part of the forefront generation creating our own way on the financial frontier. We may have our personal struggles, our moments of feeling overwhelmed, disenchanted, and even separate from the very masculine way in which money has been handled in our society as a whole up to this point. But it is so important to be gentle with ourselves, as we really don't have many role models for handling our money in an empowered feminine way. Nan eventually did learn these skills after her husband passed. She bought a house, moved across country, and began her pilgrimage on the financial frontier. In a sense, we, at any age can be new-age money priestesses, re-creating ourselves as women in the financial world, both individually and collectively.

Working with your own personal money history, just as you might examine your health history and learn more about your health, will give you the information you need to begin the unraveling of your thoughts about money and the flow of energy in your life. You can look at the areas in which you rebel, procrastinate, succumb to old paradigms and belief patterns, and maybe even give up on yourself because you are overwhelmed. I find this process of introspection to be extremely helpful and enlightening. And believe me, I have had to do some serious work around this!

MONEY AND HEALTH

I am fortunate to have the opportunity to spend some time with one of the foremost women's health gurus in the world, Dr. Christiane Northrup (author of *Women's Bodies, Women's Wisdom, The Wisdom of Menopause,* and *Mother-Daughter Wisdom*). She has been a great influence in my life and the way I work with women around overall health. As an Obstetrician/Gynecologist, she talks often about the connection between money and the second chakra*.

"Chakra" is a Sanskrit word that can be translated as "wheel" or "disk." Chakra is a concept referring to a wheel or vortex which lives along the central channel of the body. The chakras are said to be "force centers" that spin in various directions depending on their location along the midline of your body. The second chakra, located just below the navel, is all about money, power, and sex.

Interesting how the second chakra houses all three— money, sex, and power—isn't it? The way that Dr. Northrup explains is that if we are out of balance with one of these three, we will also be out of balance with the others. Therefore our money and financial health are directly related to our sexual health, both with regard to our libido and to our reproductive organ health. Our financial health is also directly connected to how empowered we feel in the world. Our financial health, or our financial stress, will eventually show up in our physical health, specifically in the reproductive and sexual areas of the body. This could manifest in ailments such as ovarian cysts, loss of sex drive, pain during sex, uterine issues, cervical health problems, and the list goes on. How interesting is that? This is why this chapter on financial health and empowerment is included in a book on health. It is one aspect of our health that we do tend to overlook even though, for many of us, it is a huge source of stress and imbalance in our lives.

Looking back to what we spoke about earlier regarding the history of money energetics and the relationship between goddess, heaven, and earth that brought us

SUE VAN RAES

abundance, I find it really interesting that imbalances in the financial area can actually rob us of our second chakra power. We, as women, intuitively know how much wisdom, intuition, and power we carry in our sexual centers, but being aware of how this part of us can be disempowered through our relationships with money—something that was originally an area over which we governed with spirit and prayer—inspires me even more to contribute to the collective healing.

Ladies, it is time to reclaim our power here—time to reclaim our responsibility as women, to hold the space for bringing back the spirituality to a part of our reality that has been stripped of the sacred. It may feel challenging on a daily basis, especially at first, but it is an important and necessary journey of healing for all of us. Imagine a world where our financial abundance and daily practices comprise an ongoing spiritual practice once again. Where when we live with purpose and integrity, financial abundance is available. This feminine energy is something the financial world needs more of. YES, we can learn a lot about money from men, and yet we also need to define money, finances, and wealth on our own terms as women.

Don't get me wrong here. I do believe there are many very relevant tools, pieces of information, systems, and experiences that are key to mastering money in your life, and that come from the more traditional, patriarchal approach to money. I am definitely not saying that we should solely chant and pray and expect everything to

184

work out. After all we are modern, educated women who can and will use our intelligence and agency in proactive ways in the contemporary world in which we live. But imagine combining spiritual knowledge, reverence, and practice with a practical, wise, and powerful money ideology. That, my dear sisters, is totally where it's at! And as an additional second-chakra benefit, just think of the orgasms that are possible when that chakra is spinning at its full potential, and in the right direction . . . the sky is the limit!!! It is time to reclaim your power with your finances. Begin the journey, and transform the blocks into bridges towards your personal health enlightenment.

THE HOW'S

Yes, this is all fine and dandy, but how do we apply these ideas to the day-to-day? How do we find our spiritual connection with money while still being real, grounded, and able to manage our day-to-day transactions and budgets?

I personally like to get help in the areas that I feel I am not well trained in. So that is just what I did around money. I found myself a financial coach, just like I would go to a therapist if I were going through a divorce, or a personal trainer if I were trying to find the right exercise routine to help me get fit. My financial coach—a woman who integrates all of these philosophies we've been examining in this chapter—is my source of support in the area of money.

Just last year, as I wrote my New Year's intentions, I realized that we women not only need to work on this individually, but also that we can be of service to each other in the world of money and finances. I requested that my financial coach put together a group of women who would meet regularly and create momentum together. We did create this group, and it was fantastic. We wove in feminine archetypes as themes to design each month around, and we looked at our beliefs, our income-generation strategies, our systems, and what we truly wanted around money. It is always helpful to band together and create a well of support with our sisters. Our next venture was a mastermind group of women who are looking to increase our income and create systems to funnel the money into different places in our lives, like savings, investments, and travel. It is so exciting, so freeing, and so empowering to work through the financial blocks while still maintaining our feminine power, which can be a huge support for success in any area, including around money.

TRANSFORMING LACK TO ABUNDANCE

Where do you fall on the spectrum of lack to abundance? When you go to your mailbox, do you cringe at the sight of the bills, or do you feel ready to manage your finances, trust in abundance, and create the balance you need with your day-to-day finances? Are you frugal like a little squirrel afraid to spend money? Or do you overspend, binge, or use retail therapy as a way to self-soothe, leaving yourself depleted and below where you need to be in your monthly budget? Do you have a budget? Know how much money you make? Or even know how much money you need to make to cover your expenses? These are all questions you will need to ask yourself in order to discover where your shadows live. As you start to unveil the patterns, the self-talk, and the ways in which you operate around money, you may be able to answer that key question: Where do you fall on the spectrum of lack to abundance, both in your thinking and in your actions?

Do you value your work, yourself, your time, and your ideas? Our abundance or lack mentality is directly proportional to how much we value ourselves. Even though money can be a source of stress for so many people, both men and women, what would it be like to feel free and inspired in your finances?

MONEY AS A SPIRITUAL PRACTICE

I have learned, as I carefully observe myself in the world of money and finances, that I do have many shadows. I avoid, I procrastinate, and I need to stay on focus with money as a daily spiritual practice. Often in the past I was met with many obstacles, but as I have moved through it, steadily, staying with the day-to-day money management techniques that I have learned, and many of which are shared in this chapter, it has gotten better. It is now easier than it used to be. My cash flow is better, my budget is more accurate, and I feel like I am better able to manifest abundance on a daily basis. I feel more "in charge" and less like I am winging it! I forecast, I move money around between different accounts, I track my spending, and I keep re-evaluating my goals around what works, what I want, and how to make that happen in my life. I recently even color-coded and re-labeled all of my files. Abundance comes in many forms, and if we can look to recognize all its shades and appearances in our lives, we learn to appreciate the good, the prosperity we do have, and the fact that we are the ones paving the way for others to feel empowered in their finances.

SYSTEMS AND STRUCTURES

There are many systems and structures that support a healthy relationship with money. Fine-tuning what works for you is a process. I find the more I can stay on top of my systems, the better. I think the first step is creating a map of intention, or a budget. Learning what your needs and expenses are each month is very helpful in setting goals and saving money.

1.   Create a budget, or map of intention

I did an exercise recently where I made 3 budgets: One for my ideal life (what I want), one for the present (what I have), and one for the lowest I could go and still make ends meet (how low can you go?). It was really helpful. I know my bottom line, and I also know what I want my income to look like to meet my ideal situation. (I share a version of this on the Health Wise website. www.HealthWise-Woman. com/healthandwealth) ♀

2.   Find a tracking system

Luckily, I recently found Mint.com. This free tracking website has been such a great tool for me to use. It sends me updates, helps me keep my budget in check with little bar graphs, reminds me of my goals and saving plans, keeps track of my credit card payments, and looks just really graphically pleasing to me overall. It is a free service that is really easy to use. Something like this can act as a great system to open our eyes to what is going on with our money situation. Any time I notice myself avoiding, up pops a reminder email from Mint.com. I know a lot of people who like Quicken or QuickBooks also, and they all have their pros and cons, but either way a tracking system of some kind is a great help. The coolest thing is that you can study how to get the most out of Mint with one of my financial gurus by just visiting the Health Wise website! Here you will learn exactly how to set Mint up and get it rockin' in your life. www.HealthWise-Woman.com/ healthandwealth ♀

3.   Create separate inspiring accounts

Creating separate accounts for different savings and periodical expense categories, as well as for a future cushion, is another great strategy. This can help you separate out goals and follow through with a plan.

I nickname my accounts for different categories I am working on building. There are some great internet banking systems that have high APYs and are easy to auto-transfer from your main account. I name them for different trips I am saving for, and it adds a little more "law of attraction" and femininity to my banking. Whatever it takes to keep you inspired and connected to your money is a good, healthy practice to include. For some of you, this may be easy, already in place, and something you have been doing for a while, but for others it may be totally new, and may even be hard to get yourself to do. Find a buddy, and help each other follow through. If you need to hire a bookkeeper, that is always an option to help you get your tracking systems set up, get organized, and move forward on your prosperity journey. Remember, empowering yourself around your finances is a critical part of your overall health.

On my most recent birthday I decided to make this entire year about Aphrodite. She is the goddess of love, passion, beauty, and sexuality. Every day I am reminded of this in my work and in my home life because I changed many account names to remind me. Every time I log into my bank account, which I now call my APHRODITE account, I remember to bring passion, inspiration, and love to my work, to my writing, and to my finances. It is interesting that it is almost six months since my last birthday, when Aphrodite came into my birthday ritual, but I am still sitting with her and her beauty every day! These little things we can do in our daily practices with our finances to remind us of what we want really can make an impact. Who, or what, are you calling in?

4.   **Add a spiritual component**

Lakshmi Practice

As we discussed earlier, the spiritual side of money can be traced throughout many cultures over the course of history, including ancient times. One of my favorite goddesses to work with is Lakshmi. She represents abundance, prosperity, and wealth. Throughout Indian history, many have prayed to her, brought her gifts, and kept shrines to her in their homes. There is even an entire day, called Lakshmi Day, dedicated to her in the Tibetan tradition. It occurs on the first new moon in November. To honor it, women light lanterns outside their homes to call in Lakshimi, offer her Prasad (gifts) of money and sweets, and chant the Lakshmi chant. The concrete part of creating abundance is important, but the spiritual side is too, and it offers a path that is about manifesting, trusting, and bringing forth your own journey to connect with deeper aspects of yourself. I want to share the Lakshmi chant with you. It is short, sweet, and very, very powerful. I use it to open my energy flow to more and more abundance.

Om-shrim-maha-lakshmi-yei-swaha

You can download an audio of the chant from my website at www.HealthWise-Woman.com/healthandwealth. I have used this chant to call in my own inner guidance, trust, and faith when I need help on the manifesting side. Lakshmi helps me to feel prosperous, supported, and connected to my own sense of inner wealth. You may be drawn to something like her, or you may have your own way of connecting to the universal force of energy through which we can manifest. Explore, open, flow. ♀

REMEMBER

Creating vibrant wealth and financial health is a whole new level of healing and empowerment. You have the ability to feel like a master of your own finances and prosperity. The combination of the practical and the spiritual sides is just magical. The femininity on the spiritual side opens up a whole new paradigm for abundance to come forth, and it can work wonders. This is how we were designed to move through our relationship to abundance. We just have to find the balance for today—the empowered modern woman's healthy approach to finances, wealth, and success. Finding alignment between your health, wealth, and womanhood in your life will have a huge impact on how you move forward, how you feel about yourself, and how you move through the world. It is at your fingertips, and all you need to do is begin the journey . . .

MEET JILL

Jill, a close friend of mine, is a 37-year-old entrepreneur in Boulder, Colorado. Jill loves yoga, being around community, being in nature, food, cooking, and sisterhood.

Living as an entrepreneur and restaurant owner in Boulder, Colorado is her passion. Jill recently co-founded SHINE, a restaurant and gathering place. She says:

"I feel abundance with both money and success, but also community and relationships that I attract. Because my work is about inspiring others, it makes me feel both generous and grateful. It also inspires me to give back in a similar way especially by supporting local business."

Jill agrees that health and happiness are very closely related: "My level of feeling abundant definitely relates to my energy during the day. When I feel in alignment with my success I feel more grounded, grateful, and confident."

Jill feels that, as a successful entrepreneur, she can feel sexy, and connected to her body. She says she often feels like dancing and expressing herself through her body, and this feeds her sense of overall strength. She also feels sexier and sassier in relationships because she can truly be herself, empowered and free.

She shares: "Fortunately, I come from a family of successful women. My grandmother was a real estate mogul, and my mom is also a successful real estate entrepreneur. Both were great mothers. Mema raised 12 kids and my mom raised us triplets and a beautiful, mentally challenged brother. I had some great role models."

Jill affirms that, through watching the models in her family, she learned that we as women can do what we want in the world. We can set our dreams as big as we want.

"In times where there are struggle, risk, and unknowns I really do rely on my spiritual practice, prosperity meditations, yoga practice—connecting inward to myself always reminds me of my inner strength. This is my feminine way of opening and allowing the natural flow of abundance in! I also surround myself with women friends that are supportive, like-minded, and inspirational and they've lifted me up and even carried me at times, and helped me remember the light and to trust the process."

Having two sisters (being one of triplets) has been an amazing gift as a constant mirror for Jill of where her money shadow lives, or any other shadow for that matter—there's nowhere for them to hide! She and her sisters always hold each other accountable with love.

She says, "I realize that we can't do it alone, but if we lean on each other as women, as community, using spirit as our inner guide, then we can continue to inspire, support and transform together, individually and as a whole. Magic happens when we are all in it together. Success is *so much more enjoyable that way, and success is about being able to share.*

It seems obvious to me that this time we are coming into is going to require us to step into our power as women, leaving a legacy for our future daughters and for womankind as a whole, but also stepping into our power, not feeling like we succumb to any stereotype. My sisters and I successfully opened our first restaurant at the age of 24, and all the odds were against us. Honestly, I felt unstoppable. Really, if the dream is there, and the belief in yourself is there, then you have essentially already created it, you just have to go do it!"

HOME PRACTICE

1. *Read and reflect upon the opening affirmation. Consider reading this or your own variation of it every morning and every night. Enjoy the benefit of the autosuggestion influencing your subconscious mind with the repetition of reading your affirmation.*

2. *Create a map of intention or monthly budget. You can use the download available on our website, or just go straight to Mint.com and use theirs. www. HealthWise-Woman.com/healthandwealth ♀*

3. *Open saving accounts of many types, put them on auto-withdrawal, and nickname them for your different goals. You can do this with your current bank, or check out INGdirect.com for an easy Internet savings account totally set up for this exact practice.*

4. *Schedule money management into your calendar. I love my FINANCE FRIDAYS. Right before the weekend, I review, update, plan ahead, and make sure things are completed and clear on the money front. What a great way to move into the weekend! Find a day and time that works for you, schedule it, write it in your calendar, follow through, and then check out how great it feels to be on top of it!*

5.   Be sure to check out special offers and connections on our website that link you directly to some of the nation's most cutting-edge success and financial coaches. Here you can check out programs and classes, and even subscribe to free newsletters to keep yourself in the woman~priestess~abundance loop. And of course check out the recording of the Lakshmi chant meditation, custom made just for the Health Wise Woman - yours to download. Have a blast!

www.HealthWise-Woman.com/healthandwealth ♀

ULTIMATE FREEDOM

SECRET # 8
The Pleasure Principle

At first it was uncomfortable, but as she began to receive love and support, her heart immediately rearranged itself to make more room for all these new good things, and just when she thought it was full, there was always room for more. Knowing this, she realized her life would never be the same again, and her heart spilled over everywhere she went.

—***Anonymous***

D id you know that there is no way to restore health and vitality to the body more quickly than by experiencing healthy pleasure? It has now been scientifically proven that good, healthy, sustainable pleasure (as opposed to the addictive, compulsive type of pleasure) is the best remedy for almost any health issue, whether chronic or acute. Given this truth, it is interesting to reflect back on the history of how pleasure has been regarded, especially for women, throughout time. It has only been in the most recent times that women have begun to restore our relationship with pleasure as part of the health and wellness conversation. We are beginning to learn and experience what actually works for us in our bodies and minds—how once we open to more joy, pleasure, and bliss, the sky is the limit on the level of pleasure we can feel. According to a study published in The National Institute of Health, research shows the role of positive emotions and pleasure, in reducing stress. Increasing positive emotions is recognized to be associated with an increase in overall quality of life, psychological well-being and physical health. In a study of young Catholic nuns dating back to the 1930's, those who experienced the most pleasure over the course of their lives lived approximately 10 years longer. Increasing our pleasure not only improves our immediate state of health, but also makes a great and tangible impact on our long-term health. We can celebrate the moment consciously, and our experience can shift with just a smile at another person, a liberating dance, a wonderful orgasm, or even a delicious piece of dark chocolate!

A BRIEF HISTORY

As discussed throughout Health Wise, there was a time when the goddess was revered as the center and essence of worship. She was held in high regard for fertility, beauty, motherhood/nurturing, and sexuality. Goddess worship dates back to the Paleolithic times, when most cultures had a matriarchal organization, and men were taught to adore, honor, and connect to both nature and the inherent power that the goddess represented. From this goddess worship extended a reverence and appreciation towards women in general. Whether she brought fertility to the land (as discussed in Secret # 7), healthy children to the tribe, healing to the sick, great pearls of wisdom to those who searched, or love and pleasure to her lover, she was held in high regard among men, among women, and within herself. Her pleasure was known as one of the most powerful healing forces known to humankind.

Eventually, feminine pleasure and the feminine principle were gradually driven out of religious worship. Women came to be seen as inferior to men, and a woman's testimony, opinion, and place in the church all became limited. Women were regarded as property, either of their father or of their husband, and their rights to personal choice and pleasure were greatly limited.

Women have fought hard to slowly regain the equality that we so deserve, but one aspect still remaining to be healed is our collective neglect of our own needs for pleasure. Women, on the whole, are known to often have so much guilt and limitation around pleasure that we constantly put all others first and forget that we will be the most radiant, healthy, vibrant, and generous individuals we can be if we actually prioritize writing our own prescriptions for pleasure.

GOOD NEWS

What would it be like to have a prescription for pleasure, confident in the knowledge that your own health would directly benefit? How would you feel knowing that your seeking out pleasure in everyday life actually increases your life span, decreases your chances for degenerative disease, and can be your spirit's way of guiding you in taking care of your health?

The best news that I have heard in the last few years is that not only do we feel good when we are granting ourselves permission for pleasure, but, as mentioned at the beginning of this chapter, it is now apparent through various clinical trials and studies that there are some drastically important health facts that support the *Pleasure Principle.* Dr. Christiane Northrup speaks frequently about this—not only the *Pleasure Principle* from a feeling sense, but also the actual biochemistry of the physiological response that occurs in our cells each time we experience pleasure

SUSTAINABLE PLEASURE

Sustainable pleasure is a form of pleasure that doesn't leave us feeling depleted, hung over, or burnt out. Sustainable pleasure directly contributes to our health in a positive way. Whether it is laughing so hard that you cry, sharing sexual intimacy with another person (or with yourself) in a safe, loving space, deep meditation or chanting, or even dancing in joy and bliss, a regular form of sustainable pleasure is critical to your health.

As many of you have likely also experienced, I have had many times in my life when I've felt guilty and even worried about being selfish when prioritizing my personal pleasure. Our culture often even gives us bonus points for being superwomen who play the martyr and put our own pleasure on the back burner. What if we could completely allow our own pleasure and passion to take the front seat?

Nitric Oxide (N.O.) is a health-promoting free radical in the body that is produced in your blood vessels. It works like this: When you experience pleasure, whether through laughter, good food, love, sexual pleasure, positive thoughts, or any other healthy, sustainable pleasure, your body releases higher levels of N.O., and this essentially allows better blood flow to circulate in your body, literally relaxing the blood vessels. N.O. even penetrates the cell walls (because it is a gas), decreasing cellular inflammation and creating better neurotransmitter function, and increasing serotonin levels and "feel-good" sensations. It has been proven that N.O. is secreted during both orgasm and conception. N.O. is the *shakti*, or the life force, or the *chi* that keeps us alive and inspired!

After almost fifteen years of mothering, and many more of being a woman, it is only recently that I can feel it in my bones that pleasure and passion are my own divine right. I know now that the better I take care of myself, the more I prioritize this necessary part of everyday health, by participating in pleasurable activities and following my passions, the better I feel, the healthier I am, and the more energy and love I have to give back to those I love.

Whether you are someone who is already good at providing yourself sustainable pleasure, or someone for whom this concept is totally foreign, the good news is, you can start right where you are. You can begin the practice of pleasure even if you have never tried it before, or if you have you can simply do it more often, heighten the pleasure you know how to have, and practice some new ways to enjoy moment-to-moment and day-to-day life. There is really never too much sustainable pleasure to be had!

PICK YOUR PLEASURES

What do you do regularly that you enjoy, that fulfills you, and that makes you feel rejuvenated, joyful, and free? This should be part of your wellness practice, so take it seriously, be creative, and be limitless. Some ideas I've previously mentioned are dance, yoga, meditation, music, art, chocolate, sex, self-pleasuring (traditionally known as masturbation), and self-massage. Other activities such as spending time in nature, aromatherapy baths, massage, facials, exercise, hugging your children, laughing, smiling at elderly women or men, dressing super wild and funky, or shoe shopping (within reason) are fun to explore. The key is to find YOUR pleasure. If this sounds like totally unfamiliar territory to you, don't despair! With just a little bit of practice and A LOT of permission from yourself, you can begin to implement the *Pleasure Principle* in your life. Start small, get comfortable, and before you know it, you will start to see the residual effects of having more pleasure, and you will never want to go back to living in guilt and shame around pleasure ever again. (Which, just as a reminder, is a good thing!)

SCHEDULE YOUR PLEASURE

I am serious! Pull out your calendar and write them down—use whatever system you normally use for scheduling, and make it happen. This is an official appointment you can have with yourself. Make it a priority. Often the culprit for us not having enough pleasure in our lives is the most common excuse in the book . . . "I don't have enough time!" The thing is, it is likely that you do have the time, but maybe not particularly good "time management." The first place to start is to look at your calendar and "find" the time. (Time is interesting that way—you can lose it, and then find it again). Eventually your pleasure time will become so important you will notice you are not forgetting it anymore, but in the beginning it is key to schedule it. We often prioritize and place a lot of importance on so many other obligations, events, appointments, etc., but we don't schedule the most precious time of all: time with ourselves! Take out your calendar, and make an appointment with yourself. You pick your pleasures, you make the time and then watch what happens!

DOUBLE YOUR PLEASURE

One of the best parts of experiencing pleasure is the fun of sharing it with someone else. Spread the pleasure vibe! Heal each other through pleasure. If you can find health and healing for you as an individual, it is pretty likely your friends, sisters, mothers, and daughters are going to start asking you what you are up to. We women like to stick together, and we don't like to miss out on much, especially something with the word "pleasure" attached (once we get over the guilt and shame conditioning, of course)! The good news about this is that you can help influence more pleasure occurring in the lives of those around you. You can be a part of healing the guilt we collectively hold around pleasure through teaching by demonstration. Last year a friend of mine and I declared an entire month "pleasure month." We gave each other full permission to indulge in our pleasures and see how amazing we could feel. Our experiment worked. We had so much fun, and thanks to Facebook and word of mouth, we inspired others around us, too. Pleasure doesn't have to cost much, or take up too much of your day, and in reality you can get refueled and become even more productive and creative in the rest of your life when you make a little time for pleasure. You don't lose anything, but you have a chance to gain everything . . .

Just as with anything else we do in our lives, can we bring awareness and equanimity to our practice of pleasure? One of the most common ways we deal with our guilt around having pleasure is by overindulging, blowing ourselves out, then letting our guilt take over and losing our inner connection with our experience of pleasure. Many of us do not get enough, so we begin to not trust ourselves in the face of pleasure, knowing we may feel out of our comfort zone and may lose control. Try making pleasure part of your regular inner practice. Try allowing it to be savored and witnessed, as a skillful practice that heightens your experience and evokes deeper consciousness, and a clearer pathway to health and happiness. Build the trust you have with yourself, and share it.

PUT SOME INTENTION INTO IT

Not only is intention heightening for the pleasure experience, but it also strengthens your mind and gives you perspective so you get to see how you respond and feel in the moment. It is like your pleasure practice is another teacher for you to learn from. This way you can watch the different sensations and thoughts that arise, and meet them with wisdom. Pleasure can be another vehicle to becoming a more integrated, more conscious individual. Have fun with this, as that is truly what it's about—joy, freedom, and love from the inside out.

MEET JESSICA

Jessica, a 26-year-old woman, is a long-time client of mine. She lives in the pristine Rocky Mountains of Colorado where she is very active with yoga, Pure Barre (a ballet-based form of exercise), and exercise. She loves movies, reading, being with her family, and designing her own jewelry.

Like many women, Jessica had a really hard time giving herself permission to have pleasure in her life. We spent many sessions working through her obstacles. Thanks to re-patterning her feelings of guilt around pleasure, Jessica has learned to include much more pleasure in her days, and has had some amazing breakthroughs around giving herself permission to do so . . .

Jessica shares: "Life is more fun when we allow different forms of pleasure. I have to recognize that I have to open to it, move through fear, and push myself, even when if feels awkward.

Having pleasure brings out the childlike joyfulness qualities that I find attractive in others. It is a quality that I want to have, have others recognize in me, and spread through example.

I want to make pleasure a priority every day, either for myself or for someone else. I am learning to find pleasure in other ways other than my old ways with food!"

Jessica has shared with me how she wants to continue to practice the Pleasure Principle and recognize when she has the opportunity to experience pleasure and let it in, without judgment or walls. She talks about her struggle with her body, her judgment of it, and how, in the past, she had measured it, grading it by what all the external influences were saying instead of listening inside.

Jessica says: "It would change hourly, daily, due to the flavor of each day, depending on the scale, how my pants fit, or simply a thought that was not supportive that I would get hooked into believing.

Embracing my femininity really helps, upping my self-care and beautifying myself.

I like the possibilities of making the most and best out of life. Giving yourself the gift of all that you deserve. Finding freedom within, freedom to have the pleasure and enjoy your body the way it is designed to be enjoyed!"

Jessica has been able to break through and experience much higher amounts of pleasure. She has worked through many challenging habits with regard to her relationship to food. She embraces being able to try new things, including discovering her sexual confidence.

Pleasure Day

On our annual women's retreat, Jessica had a major breakthrough. We spent an entire day focusing just on pleasure—diving deep into our blocks, our resistances, and our desires. Here is what happened, from Jessica's perspective:

- *"Receiving compliments was really hard, but a great exercise—I still practice that."*

- *"I could just bathe in chocolate and our chocolate pleasure meditation exercise was incredible. It keeps me mindful of my pleasure rather than rushing."*

- *"You'll never believe this! I spontaneously jumped in the pool naked, which is really unlike me! I felt proud of my spontaneity and wanted to share with the group."*

- *The icing on the cake: I surprisingly had an orgasm in the middle of the night that night in my sleep. Amazing what happens when we give ourselves permission."*

In conclusion, she says, "I am often afraid of breaking rules, getting in trouble, being too naughty or bad, or just having too much fun, but now I am seeing that the practice of having more moments infused with pleasure and breaking free into bliss is working. I feel it welling up inside me and more often I can let go and fall into pleasure . . . "

Now that is progress!!! Seeing Jessica break free and give herself permission to fully enjoy, live, and be free around our divine gift of pleasure is so inspiring. We all learn from each other.

HOME PRACTICE

1. *Schedule your pleasures: Start here: get out your calendar and find at least 3 times this week that can be your designated pleasure times. These times can be for any pleasurable activity at any time of the day, even in the evening when the house is quiet and everyone is asleep, but make sure you give yourself permission to fully experience it.*

2. *Forbidden Pleasure List: Download the Forbidden Pleasures worksheet on the Health Wise website. These are pleasures you have a hard time imagining allowing yourself to have. The sky is the limit. No guilt, no shame, no selfishness. Go for it! Then look them all over and pick two that you can actually take action toward doing. What would it take for you to complete them? Give yourself a time frame within which to experience at least two of these pleasures to the fullest. www.HealthWise-Woman.com/pleasure ♀*

3. *Chocolate Meditation: This is a great way to practice the art of pleasure as a spiritual practice. Sit down with your favorite chocolate and do a "chocolate meditation." What this means is that you experience the chocolate with every sense, slowly and mindfully. Witness the flavors, the smells, the textures, from moment to moment. If we would*

always eat chocolate like this, life would be quite different. Visit the website for a live Chocolate Meditation video!

www.HealthWise-Woman.com/pleasure ♀

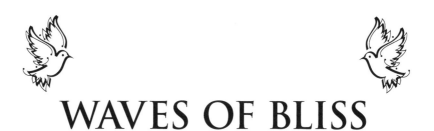

WAVES OF BLISS

If we were talking to you on your first day of physical experience, we could be of great advantage to you because we would say, "Welcome to planet Earth. There is nothing you cannot be or do or have. And your work here—your lifetime career—is to seek joy.

—Esther Hicks, channeling Abraham

If we forget, we can remember again.

— Dr. Clarissa Pinkola Estés, Ph.D.

Creating sustainable bliss, joy, and total alignment with our true selves is a continual process. We continually refine ourselves, unveiling deeper and deeper insights towards our most authentic expression in this world. It's a quest that never really ends, ceases to teach us valuable life lessons, or rests in one place for any length of time. With that said, there often comes a time when we realize that something is working to our benefit. There is that moment when we see the results from all the diligence of our personal work and awareness supporting us in our overall health, happiness, and self-love. We sort out what our way is on this magical ride.

Riding the waves of bliss is how I describe the process of noticing how our lives have evolved as a whole, whilst meeting our challenges with a wiser, more seasoned, and more centered, approach. We trust ourselves more, and we are able to live in the moment more fully. Our cars still break down, we still lose jobs, get sick, and sometimes even go through life's inevitable heartbreaks. All of these colorful and challenging moments are still looking us right in the eye—the difference is, now we have a well of inner strength and love that guides us more gracefully to the most centered path.

I was in a yoga class the other day and the teacher spoke of grace. "Grace" is a commonly used word, and in one particular style of Yoga, there is a foundational principle called "opening to grace." In this class, the teacher explained that, in the beginning of any spiritual practice, we strive to feel this grace, and we strive to even allow and open to the grace that we inherently are, but as we deepen our practice (whatever that may be), become more attuned to ourselves, our breath, and the infusion of love into our lives, we can begin to tap into grace in its fullest form. This is exactly what happens as we create alignment in our health, body, mind, and relationships, and start to feel the beauty that we are. We tap into grace in our lives. We ride the waves of bliss each day with ever-deeper surrender, knowing that in order to experience bliss and happiness, we must enjoy each moment, without attachment.

Eventually, we feel that our lives have come more into balance, and we have a sense that we have arrived, so to speak. We become most at home in ourselves, achieving a sort of paradise within that is untouchable by any external event, even a really hard one.

I know you all have moments of this. This process is really about bringing into our life experience more and more healthful moments so that riding our inner waves of bliss becomes a practice in and of itself.

As we have touched upon previously, there are ways in which we are conditioned to self-sabotage, question ourselves, complain, and even to keep wanting more and more without ever settling into a moment of contentment. Sitting with contentment is a beautiful part of the practice. Staying present, finding gratitude for the moment, and celebrating ourselves are all great ways to stay connected and remind ourselves to savor the moment when the waves of bliss do show up.

SAVORING THE MOMENT

Just as we practiced in our chocolate meditation, savoring the moment through the senses is a helpful way to stay connected to gratitude and bliss. The senses are our connection to the present and, tuning into them heightens the pleasure we experience in each moment. Savoring the moment is a huge gift to ourselves. We can literally watch time slow down, thereby experiencing more optimal health and deeper attunement with ourselves. We can make beauty shine all around us from the inside out, and share it with others. We allow our hearts to swell with love, and that opens us more deeply than anything else. We will forget, and then remember again—that is human. We tune out and then we tune back in. The forgetting and remembering are almost like the rhythm of each breath, or the rhythm of each wave. Each time the remembering is easier, and each time we are more connected to our bliss, both within and without. We learn to open to infinite possibilities, feel the vibrancy of our bodies, love more deeply, and find beauty in the moment-to-moment experience of living!

SUE VAN RAES

LIVE GRATITUDE

Last year, on Thanksgiving of all days, I drew a card from my favorite Tarot deck, the Crowley deck. The card (6 of cups) signified "pleasure," which was an interesting message to receive on Thanksgiving. As I read further, and thought more about the reading, I began to really understand the mystical significance of pulling this card on this Thanksgiving Day. The indication, or meaning, of the card read: "The best way to express your gratitude in each moment is through pleasure." What a perfect card for that day.

There are many ways to express gratitude and make it into a practice. Here are a few of my favorites:

1.   **Thank You Mantra** Speaking the works "THANK YOU" is harder than it sounds. Observe yourself when you receive a compliment, recognition, praise, or acknowledgement! For many of us it is hard to receive and take it in. Can you acknowledge the gratitude through a "thank you" more often? It may seem insignificant, but it is a powerful shift of awareness to bring in.

2.   **Three Questions** Each day, ask yourself three questions to bring yourself into a state of gratitude. (This is great to include in your morning meditation.):

- How can I take care of myself today?

- What am I thankful for today?

- How can I share my gifts more fully in the world today?

3.   **Create a Gratitude Vision Board** Using your favorite photos, magazines, funky paper, poetry, etc., create a gratitude vision board that reflects all that you are grateful for in your life. Not only is this a major "thank you" out loud, but it is also a magnet that can attract more and more to be thankful for. This exercise is really fun and will up the ante of your gratitude game!

Riding the waves of bliss is a way to acknowledge the beauty in each moment, whether simple or grandiose. We can make the ordinary extraordinary. This is an important part of living life to the fullest. All the work we do in our lives to be mindful, in balance, and on track with what we want deserves a moment of witnessing. We can celebrate our successes, and see to all that we have created. Our souls crave acknowledgement, joy, and gratitude in order for us to be fulfilled in our personal quests.

As you continue the personal revolution in your own life, may it be filled with exactly what you need to cultivate your truth in this world. May you be happy, may you be healthy, and may you find joy in sharing yourself with others.

True health continues to be a teacher for each of us, meeting us exactly where we are, each moment of each day. May we awaken to life as our teacher, listen inward, and open to inner bliss as each of our unique ventures brings us together in this great collective mission to shift the paradigm for women as a whole.

Shine on sisters . . . I will always continue to be your humble student.

I'd love to hear your stories and feedback, and to know more about who my readers are. Please feel free to email me anytime and visit: www.HealthWise-Woman.com for endless resources, community, and connection . . . we are in this together! ♀

In divine health and gratitude,

Sue

Our deepest fear is not that we are inadequate.
Our deepest fear is that we are powerful beyond measure.
It is our light, not our darkness that frightens us most.
We ask ourselves, 'Who am I to be brilliant, gorgeous,
talented, and famous?'
Actually, who are you not to be?
You are a child of God.
Your playing small does not serve the world.
There is nothing enlightened about shrinking so that people
won't feel insecure around you.
We were born to make manifest the glory of God that is
within us.
It's not just in some of us; it's in all of us.
And when we let our own light shine, we unconsciously give
other people permission to do the same.
As we are liberated from our own fear, our presence
automatically liberates others.

—Marianne Williamson

HEALTH WISE

True Health and Happiness for the Empowered Woman

Health Wise and the work of Sue Van Raes is designed for women of all ages seeking to live their best selves. The passionate mission Sue intends is to support women to learn through understanding and knowing their own personal bodies, while listening to their intuition, internal rhythm, and wisdom. Sue works with clients individually, leads virtual groups, and international retreats worldwide. She also speaks to groups of women around the country who are seeking inspiration and support in their own process toward greater health and happiness.

Please visit our interactive website where you can find more resources, connect with other women, and go deeper into your own personal passion for living. There are many wonderful tools, worksheets, videos, live interviews and audio tracks to interact with there.
www.HealthWise-Woman.com ♀

To stay connected to upcoming events with Health Wise community and be a part of our mailing list please visit

www.HealthWise-Woman.com ♀

www.BoulderNutrition.com

Or visit us on Facebook at **Health Wise Woman**